Diagnosing and Managing Headaches

Second Edition

Seymour Diamond, MD

Diamond Headache Clinic
Inpatient Headache Unit,
Columbus Hospital
Chicago, Illinois

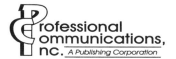

Professional Communications, Inc. *A Publishing Corporation*

Published by:
Professional Communications, Inc.

For orders, please call:
1-800-337-9838

ISBN: 1-884735-27-4

Printed in the United States of America

This text is printed on recycled paper.

DEDICATION

To Elaine, for caring.

ACKNOWLEDGMENT

I would like to express my appreciation to Mary A. Franklin and Phyllis Jones Freeny for their invaluable editorial assistance in the completion of this book. Also, thanks to Nikki D. Stewart for proofreading and typography.

ABOUT THE AUTHOR

Dr. Seymour Diamond is Director of the Diamond Headache Clinic and the Inpatient Headache Unit, Columbus Hospital, Chicago, Illinois. He is adjunct Professor of Pharmacology and Molecular Biology, The Chicago Medical School, North Chicago, Illinois. He serves the National Headache Foundation as Executive Director.

TABLE OF CONTENTS

TABLES

FIGURES

Introduction

It has been estimated that from 60 to 70 million Americans have experienced some form of headache. This universal problem has prompted the National Institutes of Health to conduct epidemiological surveys to determine the populations affected by headache and its impact on the economy. In a survey of 15,000 households in Washington County, Maryland, 10,169 residents between the ages of 12 to 29 years responded to specific questions about headaches. Of this group, 57.1% of the males and 76.5% of the females experienced a headache in the previous 4 weeks. Four or more headaches in the prior month were described by 6.1% of the males and 14.0% of the females. If these data hold true for the rest of the nation, headache is one of the most prevalent problems to be confronted by the practicing physician.

Many headache sufferers will not consult a physician for the occasional tension-type headache. However, it is estimated that over 4 billion dollars are spent annually on over-the-counter remedies for headache pain. If we add the monies spent on prescription drugs, the expense of lost workdays, fees for numerous visits to physicians' offices and emergency departments, and repeated hospitalizations, the fiscal impact is staggering.

For the physician treating the patient with headaches, it is essential to be aware of the various causes of this problem. The physician should always be alert for the patient presenting with recent onset of headaches—a signal that a careful workup is needed to rule-out organic, and possibly morbid, causes for the headache problem.

To effectively treat the patient with headache, an accurate diagnosis must be established. A headache history is important in evaluating the patient with headaches. A complete and thorough physical and neurological examination will facilitate the diagnosis, and the physician should be cognizant of the specific diagnostic tests used in headache workups. Finally, the clinician should be aware that adequate preventive therapy is available for patients and s/he is not limited to prescribing pain relief measures.

The purpose of this text is to serve as a reference for the practitioner who will encounter headache patients more frequently than anticipated. The book is enhanced by flow charts to assist the physician in establishing the diagnosis and selecting the appropriate therapy.

Resources for the Physician

The physician treating headache patients has two major resources in the United States. The National Headache Foundation (NHF) is the oldest and largest organization for the headache patients, their families and friends, and their treating physicians. The NHF serves as a resource center and supports education through public seminars held throughout the United States. To further research into the diagnosis and treatment of headache, the NHF provides grants for a variety of investigations. The physician members are listed in the professional membership directory and included on the state list of physician members. They receive professional and lay educational material, quarterly newsletters for distribution to their patients, professional discounts, and grant considerations. For further information, contact:

National Headache Foundation
428 West St. James Place, 2nd Floor
Chicago, IL 60614
Telephone: 1-800-843-2256
Fax: 1-773-525-7357

The physician interested in the treatment of headache and the continuing research into this problem may be interested in joining a professional organization, The American Association for the Study of Headaches (AASH). For information regarding this organization, founded in 1959, contact:

AASH Headquarters
875 Kings Highway, Suite 200
Woodbury, NJ 08096
Telephone: 1-609-845-0322
Fax: 1-609-384-5811

REFERENCES

1. Diamond S, Dalessio DJ. *The Practicing Physician's Approach to Headache*, 5th ed. Diamond S, Dalessio DJ (eds). Baltimore: Williams & Wilkins; 1992.

2. Linet MS, Stewart WF, Celentano DD, Ziegler D, Sprecher M. An epidemiologic study of headache among adolescents and young adults. *JAMA*. 1989;261:2211-2216.

1   Classification and Etiology

To facilitate establishing the diagnosis, an understanding of the classification of the various headache types is essential. The Ad Hoc Committee of the National Institutes of Health undertook this rigorous task with the first extensive classification system of headache. In 1988, the International Headache Society developed comprehensive classification and diagnostic criteria.

For the sake of clarity, a simple classification table is used (Table 1.1). In this system, headaches are divided into three major categories:
- Vascular
- Tension-type (muscle contraction)
- Traction and inflammatory.

Vascular Headache

Common to all types of vascular headache is a tendency to vascular dilation which precipitates the headache phase. The vascular dilation is due to various triggers including:
- Menses
- Fever
- Stress
- Weather
- Altitude
- Foods containing vasoactive substances and vasodilators such as the nitrates.

Vascular headaches include:
- Migraine (with or without aura)
- Cluster

TABLE 1.1 — CLASSIFICATION OF HEADACHES

Vascular
- Migraine
  - With aura
  - Without aura
- Complicated hemiplegic
- Ophthalmoplegic basilar artery
- Cluster
- Toxic vascular
- Hypertensive

Tension-type
- Depressive equivalents and conversion reactions
- Chronic anxiety states
- Cervical osteoarthritis
- Chronic myositis

Traction and Inflammatory
- Mass lesions (tumors, edema, hematomas, cerebral hemorrhage)
- Diseases of the eye, ear, nose, throat and teeth
- Arteritis, phlebitis and cranial neuralgia
- Occlusive vascular disease
- Atypical facial pain
- Temporomandibular joint (TMJ) disorder

Adapted from: Diamond S, Dalessio DJ. Classification and mechanism(s) of headache. In: *The Practicing Physician's Approach to Headache*, 5th ed. Diamond S, Dalessio DJ (eds). Baltimore: Williams & Wilkins; 1992:1-10.

- Toxic vascular headache
- Hypertensive headache.

Tension-type Headaches

Tension-type headaches are characterized by the "muscle contraction" which occurs with these headaches. This category can be further divided into:
- Episodic
- Chronic.

Most people experiencing episodic tension-type headaches will use simple, over-the-counter analgesics to obtain relief. Chronic tension-type headaches are usually linked to depression or anxiety. The majority of patients seeking a physician's help with their headaches is experiencing chronic tension-type headaches.

Traction and Inflammatory Headaches

Headache due to organic disease is classified as traction and inflammatory headache. The causes of these headaches include:
- Mass lesions such as:
  - Brain tumors
  - Hematomas
  - Cerebral hemorrhage
  - Cerebral edema
- Arteritis
- Phlebitis
- Cranial neuralgia
- Temporomandibular joint (TMJ) disorder.

These types of headaches may have morbid consequences. Management is dependent on the etiology, and immediate treatment may be indicated.

A headache diagnostic guide is provided to facilitate diagnosis in a clear, concise manner (Table 1.2). A thorough headache history and appropriate diagnostic testing will aid in confirmation of the diagnosis.

TABLE 1.2 — HEADACHE DIAGNOSTIC GUIDE

	Migraine	Cluster	Tension-type (Chronic)	Mass Lesion
Frequency	2 to 8/month	1 to 3/day during a series	Daily or almost daily	Varied
Duration	4 hours to 2 days, usually 12 to 18 hours	30 to 90 minutes	Constant	Varied
Onset	Gradual	Sudden, reaches peak of intensity in 1 to 3 minutes	Gradual	Varied, though onset of complaint may have been recent
Pain area	Unilateral, may switch sides or become bilateral	Unilateral, usually retro-orbital	Hatband, bilateral	Unilateral
Characteristic pain	Throbbing, pulsating; moderate to severe	Steady, severe, excruciating, knife-like, sharp, probing	Steady, dull ache	Varied

Associated symptoms	Systemic–usually nausea or vomiting, prodrome in migraine with aura, premonitory signs in migraine without aura	Ipsilateral symptoms, partial Horner's syndrome	None	Varied
Triggers	Stress, menses, alcohol, food additives	During a series, alcohol will trigger attack	Stress	None known
Sex distribution	3:1 female	10:1 male	Equal distribution	Equal distribution

REFERENCES

Ad Hoc Committee. Classification of headache. *JAMA*. 1962;6:717.

Headache Classification Committee of the International Headache Society. Classification and diagnostic criteria for headache disorders, cranial neuralgias and facial pain. *Cephalalgia*. 1988;8(suppl 7):1-96.

2   Diagnosis

History

Obtaining a complete headache history is the most vital tool in the diagnosis and management of the headache patient (Figure 2.1). Certain items should be included on the headache history to simplify this process:

- Type of headache
- Onset
- Frequency
- Site
- Duration
- Severity and character
- Prodromata
- Associated symptoms
- Precipitating factors
- Sleep pattern
- Emotional factors
- Family history
- Medical, surgical or obstetrical history
- Allergy
- Previous medications and therapies
- Present medications.

■ Types of Headache

It is important to determine if the patient is experiencing more than one type of headache. Some patients with a long history of recurrent, one-sided, severe headaches will note a milder, daily headache. The patient may also note a change in headache pattern, which could alert the physician to a serious etiology.

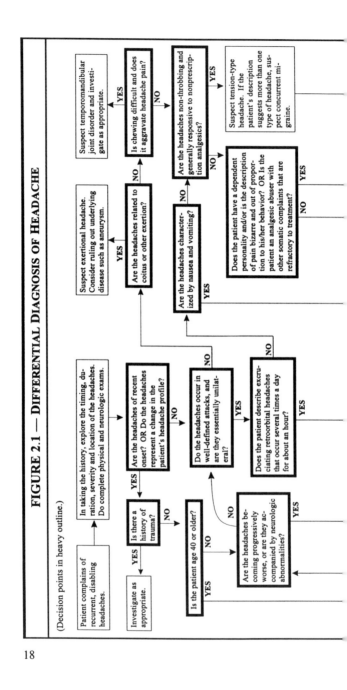

FIGURE 2.1 — DIFFERENTIAL DIAGNOSIS OF HEADACHE

(Decision points in heavy outline.)

Patient complains of recurrent, disabling headaches.

In taking the history, explore the timing, duration, severity and location of the headaches. Do complete physical and neurologic exams.

Is there a history of trauma?

YES → Investigate as appropriate.

NO → Are the headaches of recent onset? OR Do the headaches represent a change in the patient's headache profile?

YES → Is the patient age 40 or older?

YES

NO → Are the headaches becoming progressively worse, or are they accompanied by neurologic abnormalities?

YES / NO

NO → Do the headaches occur in well-defined attacks, and are they essentially unilateral?

YES → Does the patient describe excruciating retroorbital headaches that occur several times a day for about an hour?

YES

NO → Are the headaches characterized by nausea and vomiting?

YES → Are the headaches related to coitus or other exertion?

YES → Suspect exertional headache. Consider ruling out underlying disease such as aneurysm.

NO → Is chewing difficult and does it aggravate headache pain?

YES → Suspect temporomandibular joint disorder and investigate as appropriate.

NO → Are the headaches non-throbbing and generally responsive to nonprescription analgesics?

YES → Suspect tension-type headache. If the patient's description suggests more than one type of headache, suspect concurrent migraine.

NO

NO → Does the patient have a dependent personality and/or is the description of pain bizarre and out of proportion to his/her behavior? OR Is the patient an analgesic abuser with other somatic complaints that are refractory to treatment?

YES / NO

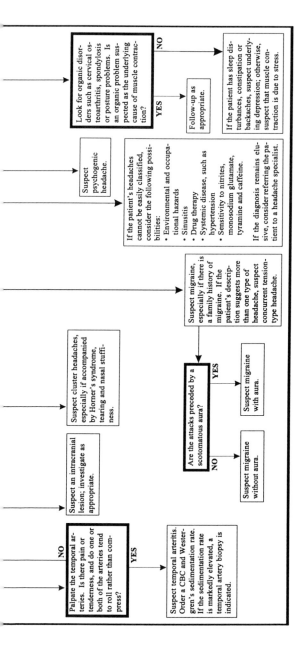

Palpate the temporal arteries. Is there pain or tenderness, and do one or both of the arteries tend to roll rather than compress?

NO

YES

Suspect temporal arteritis. Order a CBC and Westergren's sedimentation rate. If the sedimentation rate is markedly elevated, a temporal artery biopsy is indicated.

Suspect an intracranial lesion; investigate as appropriate.

Suspect cluster headaches, especially if accompanied by Horner's syndrome, tearing and nasal stuffiness.

Are the attacks preceded by a scotomatous aura?

YES

Suspect migraine with aura.

NO

Suspect migraine without aura.

Suspect migraine, especially if there is a family history of migraine. If the patient's description suggests more than one type of headache, suspect concurrent tension-type headache.

Suspect psychogenic headache.

If the patient's headaches cannot be easily classified, consider the following possibilities:
• Environmental and occupational hazards
• Sinusitis
• Drug therapy
• Systemic disease, such as hypertension
• Sensitivity to nitrites, monosodium glutamate, tyramine and caffeine.

If the diagnosis remains elusive, consider referring the patient to a headache specialist.

Look for organic disorders such as cervical osteoarthritis, spondylosis or posture problems. Is an organic problem suspected as the underlying cause of muscle contraction?

YES

Follow-up as appropriate.

NO

If the patient has sleep disturbances, constipation or backaches, suspect underlying depression; otherwise, suspect that muscle contraction is due to stress.

2

■ Onset

Determining the age of onset of the headaches may provide a significant clue to the type of headache the patient is experiencing. Migraine headaches usually start in adolescence or the early twenties. Patients with cluster headaches will usually describe headache onset in their third, fourth or fifth decade. The patient with tension-type headaches will note that the headaches started during their thirties or forties. The physician should rule out organic disease in those patients whose headaches start after age 50.

The patient should also be questioned regarding any specific event which may have precipitated the headache onset, such as:

- Following some type of:
  - Trauma
  - Infection
- Female patients relating onset:
  - At menarche
  - During pregnancy
  - At menopause.

■ Frequency

Frequency of the headache attacks not only provides a clue to the diagnosis but will also impact on the type of treatment selected. Migraine typically occurs 2 to 8 times per month. Chronic tension-type headaches are characterized by their daily occurrence. The patient with cluster headaches will describe a series of headaches, occurring a few times per day for several weeks, and then disappearing for months or years. The headache associated with organic disease may not demonstrate a particular pattern and may be progressive in frequency as well as other features.

■ Site

Migraine is typically a one-sided headache, although it may occur bilaterally and may switch sides.

Unilateral headaches are also indicative of organic disease. Cluster headaches are typically one-sided and do not switch sides during a series of headaches. The tension-type headache is notably bilateral and the pain may be described as a tight band around the head (hatband). Patients may also note pain radiating to the neck and shoulder.

■ **Duration**

An acute migraine attack usually continues from 4 to 24 hours. However, some patients will experience their headaches for 2 or more days, and may be classified as suffering from status migraine. Cluster headaches are noted for their brief duration, lasting from a few minutes to 3 or 4 hours. The pain associated with trigeminal neuralgia is described as short jabs, lasting a few seconds. Tension-type headaches are continuous, with occasional variations in severity.

■ **Severity and Character**

The pain of migraine is severe, may be incapacitating, and is described as throbbing or pulsating. Cluster headache pain is depicted as excruciating pain and may be throbbing or depicted as deep and boring pain. Chronic, tension-type headaches are persistent, dull, aching or vise-like. In the headache due to organic causes, the pain is progressive in nature and intensity.

■ **Prodromata**

Migraine is classified according to the presence of warning symptoms or aura. Migraine with aura is characterized by the appearance of warning signs 30 to 60 minutes before the onset of headache symptoms. These symptoms are usually neurological in nature. More severe neurological symptoms, such as ocular paralysis or hemiparesis, may occur with complicated migraine. Premonitory signs, such as intense hunger, fatigue or bursts of energy, may precede an acute attack of migraine with or without aura. Visual symptoms, such as teichopsia (fortification spectrum), may occur with headache due to tumor or angioma.

■ Associated Symptoms

The presence of associated symptoms may also provide clues to the diagnosis. Migraine symptoms include:

- A "sick headache" due to accompanying gastrointestinal (GI) symptoms such as:
  - Nausea
  - Vomiting
- Dizziness
- Photo- and/or phonophobia
- Tinnitus
- Blurred vision.

Cluster headache is also characterized by its associated symptoms such as:

- Lacrimation
- Facial flushing
- Nasal congestion
- A partial Horner's syndrome.

The headache due to organic causes may also occur in association with:

- Double vision
- Seizures
- Tinnitus.

Patients suffering from chronic, tension-type headaches often provide the treating physician with long lists of somatic, emotional and psychic symptoms.

■ Precipitating Factors

An inventory of precipitating factors associated with acute headache attacks may help:

- Determine the diagnosis
- In preventing the headaches.

Migraine can be triggered by a variety of precipitants such as:

- Diet
- Oversleeping
- Fatigue
- Menstruation
- Changes in weather and barometric pressure
- Foods containing vasoactive substances
- Certain drugs, including:
  - Nitroglycerine
  - Indomethacin.

Stress may trigger any type of headache, and migraine patients will note that an acute migraine attack may occur in a let-down period. During a cluster series, alcohol may precipitate an acute attack, although the patient will not note a relationship outside a cluster period. In patients who relate headache to exertion or straining, the physician should be suspicious of organic causes, although benign exertional factors may be the mechanism.

■ Sleep Pattern

The patient presenting with headache should be questioned about any sleep disturbances. Cluster patients will often note that headaches will awaken them at the same time each night during a cluster series. In migraine patients, the headaches are often present when the patient awakens. Patients with chronic, tension-type headaches will often relate early or frequent awakening. These sleep disturbances may be a manifestation of depression. In headaches due to anxiety, the patient will complain of difficulty falling asleep. Hypertensive headache is characterized by its presence upon awakening and its gradual diminishing during the day. Headache due to acute sinusitis will not be present early in the morning but will increase during the day.

■ Emotional Factors

When obtaining a headache history, the physician should question the patient about family, marital and work relationships. Stressors related to the patient's home or work life can greatly impact on the headache pattern. Because the patient may not feel comfortable with the interviewer during the initial visit, these questions may need to be addressed during later visits.

■ Family History

Migraine is a familial disorder, and most patients will relate a family history of similar headaches. Cluster headache patients will not relate a family history of headaches. In patients with chronic, tension-type headaches, a family history of depression may also be reported.

■ Medical, Surgical and/or Obstetrical History

The patient's previous history may impact on diagnosis and possible therapy. The physician should determine any prior incidence of head trauma. The patient should also be questioned regarding any previous neurosurgeries or lumbar punctures. Migraine patients may note a decrease or remission of headaches during pregnancy.

■ Allergy

The patient may relate the headaches to specific allergies or sensitivities to foods. A seasonal relationship is noted in cluster headaches with frequent occurrences in spring and fall.

■ **Previous Medications and Therapies**

The patient with chronic headaches may produce an extensive list of previously tried drugs. They have often undergone various tests and consulted several physicians. Determining the success or failures of previous therapies may assist in diagnosing the headaches or selecting appropriate treatments.

2

■ **Present Medications**

The physician must inventory the medications the patient is currently using. Certain drugs may trigger headaches such as:

- Nitrates
- Reserpine
- Indomethacin
- Minoxidil
- Apresoline.

Female patients using oral contraceptives or postmenopausal hormones may note an increase in the severity, frequency, duration or complications of their migraine attacks.

Physical, Neurological and Diagnostic Workup

A thorough physical and neurological examination is essential to rule out organic pathology for the headaches, as well as determine which diagnostic tests are required. Simple observation of the patient during the interview process will provide many clues to the physician. A person with an acute severe headache, whether it is organic or vascular in etiology, may walk and move slowly and deliberately to avoid jarring which often intensifies the pain. A patient who presents with a calm and relaxed demeanor although complaining of a severe, disabling headache may be

suffering from headaches due to depression. The vasomotor instability of migraine may manifest as:
- Blotching of the skin on the chest
- Sweaty palms
- Occasionally, urticaria.

■ **Physical Workup**
  The physical examination should include:
  - Vital signs
    - Fever may be indicative of systemic infection. In the presence of neck stiffness, meningitis must be ruled out.
    - Hypertensive headache occurs with diastolic pressures of 110 mm Hg or higher.
    - Rapid pulse is indicative of vasomotor instability.
  - Examination of the head
    - Palpation and auscultation
    - Prominent temporal artery may be indicative of:
      - Temporal arteritis, or
      - An acute migraine attack.
  - Examination of the eyes
    - Characteristics of cluster headaches include:
      - Partial Horner's syndrome
      - Lacrimation
      - Conjunctival injection
      - Unilateral ptosis.
    - Tonometry should be performed on patients over age 40 to rule out glaucoma.
  - Examination of ears and nose (rule out infection or disease).
  - Examination of the face (presence of trigger points is indicative of trigeminal neuralgia).
  - Examination of the neck (limitation of motion, spasm and tenderness should be evaluated).

Neurological examination should include:
- Systemic examination of the cranial nerves
- Evaluation of motor function
- Sensory testing
- Tests of coordination
  - Evaluate gait
  - Finger-to-nose and heel-to-shin tests
  - Romberg test.

Diagnostic testing may be required to rule out organic causes of the headache and establish a baseline of some parameters although many headache patients have undergone previous testing. Repeat testing may be required if the patient's headache pattern has changed suddenly or if prior results were questionable. Invasive testing should be avoided, if possible, as these tests may increase the patient's headaches or cause more severe complications. Diagnostic testing should include:
- Neuroimaging, including:
  - Computed tomography (CT) scan
  - Magnetic resonance imaging (MRI)
  - Magnetic resonance angiography (MRA)
- Lumbar puncture
- Electroencephalogram (EEG)
- Other diagnostic tests.

■ Neuroimaging
If the physician is not confident in the diagnosis, or if certain aspects of the history suggest possible organic causes of the headache, neuroimaging should be considered. The *Standards of Care* of the National Headache Foundation have established guidelines to determine if neuroimaging is indicated (Table 2.1).

Little conclusive evidence is available to recommend one procedure over the other. However, certain exceptions should be noted when ordering these procedures:

TABLE 2.1 — GUIDELINES FOR USE OF CT AND MRI

The use of neuroimaging procedures may be indicated when *any* of the following is present:
- Decreased alertness or cognition
- Onset of pain with exertion, coitus, coughing or sneezing
- Worsening under observation
- Nuchal rigidity
- Focal neurological signs
- First headache in patient over age 50
- Worst headache ever experienced
- Headache not fitting a defined pattern.

The use of neuroimaging procedures *may not* be indicated when *all* of the following are present:
- History of similar headaches
- Normal vital signs
- Alertness and cognition intact
- Supple neck
- No neurological signs
- Improvement in headache without analgesics or abortive medications.

Abbreviations: CT, computed tomography; MRI, magnetic resonance imaging.

Adapted from: National Headache Foundation. *Standards of Care for Headache Diagnosis and Treatment.* Chicago, Ill: National Headache Foundation; 1996:6-7.

- CT scan without contrast for detection of subarachnoid hemorrhage
- MRI for detection of posterior fossa disease as manifested by exertional-, coital-, cough-, or sneeze-induced headache
- MRI in conjunction with MRA for visualization of aneurysm or other vascular lesion.

CT Scan

CT scanning has precluded the use of hazardous invasive testing. For the headache patient, the CT scan will aid in ruling out disorders that can produce chronic headache:

- Brain tumors
- Chronic subdural hematoma
- Hydrocephalus.

Because CT scanning can be performed during an acute migraine attack, this test has identified transient morphologic changes after an acute headache, including edema in the cerebral parenchyma. Abnormalities may be demonstrated in CT scans of patients experiencing complicated migraine (such as transient cerebral edema). Cerebral ventricle enlargement and cerebral cortical atrophy may be observed in patients with repeated severe attacks.

Magnetic Resonance Imaging

Magnetic resonance imaging has greatly enhanced the physician's capabilities in determining occult causes of headaches. MRI can identify lesions that were previously impossible to visualize. This type of imaging can be done in the frontal, sagittal or the axial projections. An important difference between MRI and CT scanning is that CT scanning uses x-rays which produce denser images. However, MRI measures the physical and physiological functions within brain tissue and can then differentiate various normal structures as well as pathological tissues. MRI can also detect certain abnormalities at a very early stage, thus allowing for prompt treatment. Because MRI can differentiate white and gray matter within the brain, it can demonstrate several disorders:

- Demyelinizing plaques, such as those seen in multiple sclerosis
- Brain tumors

- Strokes
- Brainstem and posterior fossa lesions
- Spinal cord abnormalities
- Herniated intervertebral discs.

If an abnormality of the brain or spinal cord is suspected, MRI should be performed. The procedure can be accomplished without the injection of dye in sensitive patients, and the risk of radiation is absent. Although the majority of headache patients do not need to be evaluated with this procedure, it does offer an excellent tool in ruling out organic disorders.

Magentic Resonance Angiography
Magnetic resonance angiography can be useful in those patients in whom there is suspicion of a vascular abnormality.

■ Lumbar Puncture
This invasive procedure should only be undertaken if the symptoms warrant. A patient presenting with fever and neck stiffness should undergo a lumbar puncture to rule out intracranial infection. Because herniation of the brainstem into the foramen magnum can occur if spinal fluid is removed suddenly in the presence of a brain tumor, lumbar puncture should be avoided until other diagnostic procedures are performed.

The risk of post-spinal headache should be considered before attempting lumbar puncture or spinal anesthesia. This type of headache is described in Chapter 8, *Post-traumatic Headache*.

■ Electroencephalogram
The EEG is not used extensively because of the availability and efficiency of other tests. This test is indicated in patients presenting with headache accom-

panied by seizure. Its results are inconclusive in most patients with chronic headache.

■ Other Diagnostic Tests

Obtaining baseline values for blood chemistries, CBC and urinalysis will assist the physician in continuing therapy for the headache patient. Hypothyroidism has been noted to cause headache and T_3 and T_4 should be obtained at the initial visit. A sedimentation rate by Westergren's method should be obtained on all patients over age 50 with recent onset of headache to rule out temporal arteritis.

For patients receiving β-blocker or calcium channel blocker therapy, a baseline electrocardiogram (EKG) is essential. With continued therapy, review of laboratory values should be performed periodically to determine if there has been any change due to therapy. With certain medications (eg, lithium), serum levels must be evaluated to determine dosages.

REFERENCES

Davidoff RA. *Migraine: Manifestations, Pathogenesis, and Management*. Philadelphia, Pa: FA Davis Co; 1995.

Diamond S, Dalessio DJ (eds). *The Practicing Physician's Approach to Headache*, 5th ed. Baltimore, Md: Williams & Wilkins; 1992.

Evans RW. Diagnostic testing for the evaluation of headaches. *Neurol Clin*. 1996;14:1-26.

National Headache Foundation. *Standards of Care for Headache Diagnosis and Treatment*. Chicago, Ill: National Headache Foundation; 1996;6-7.

Prager JM, Rosenblum J, Mikulis DJ, Diamond S, Freitag FG. Evaluation of headache patients by MRI. *Headache Q*. 1991;2:192-195.

3

Headaches Due to Organic Causes

The classification of organic headache includes headache due to:
- Space occupying lesion
- Infection
- Low cerebrospinal fluid (CSF) pressure
- Cranial arteritis
- Major neuralgias.

As with other types of headache, diagnosis is based on:
- History
- Physical examination
- Laboratory results
- Radiologic examinations.

All patients must undergo careful and thorough examinations to rule out these possibly morbid causes. Selection of therapy is totally dependent on the cause of the headaches.

Physicians should always be alert to recent onset of headaches starting in a patient age 40 or older. They should also be vigilant in evaluating the patient who has experienced a recent change in a headache pattern that had been consistent for many years. The physician should also be wary of the presentation of recent onset of headache in a patient with a prior history of cancer.

A headache produced by an intracranial lesion is usually attributed to:
- Inflammation
- Traction

- Displacement of the pain-sensitive structures of the head, most often the blood vessels.

The term "traction headache" is based on the displacement of these structures as a result of traction.

The following pattern is demonstrated in headaches resulting from intracranial lesions:

- A steady, non-throbbing, deep, dull ache
- The headache can awaken the patient from a sound sleep
- The headache is intermittent, although it can be continuous in some patients
- The headache is rarely as intense as the headache associated with fever
- Exertion can trigger or exacerbate the headache
- The frequency and duration will progressively increase.

Tumor

Headache is always a cardinal sign of rapidly increasing intracranial pressure. However, a slow growing tumor may cause a dull, transitory headache that is relieved by simple analgesics. Some generalizations can be made about headache due to brain tumor:

- In about one third of patients with headache due to brain tumor, the pain overlies the tumor. However, in the remaining patients, the headache may be referred from a distant intracranial source.
- A tumor below the tentorium will frequently cause occipital pain and cervical muscle spasm.
- A tumor above the tentorium will often manifest as a headache at the vertex or in the frontal regions.
- If the tumor is at the midline, exertion such as coughing, straining or sudden head movement can exacerbate the headache.

- A tumor that is chiasmal at the sella may cause the pain to be referred to the vertex.
- A posterior fossa tumor usually manifests as a headache.
- If the tumor is hemispheric, the headache is usually felt on the ipsilateral side.
- A lesion in the pituitary fossa often causes a frontal and bitemporal headache, which is bursting in character.
- Pain is often present behind the ear in a cerebellopontine angle lesion.

Headache rarely occurs as an initial symptom with several lesions, such as craniopharyngiomas and hypophysial adenomas. However, it can be an initial manifestation with other tumors, such as:

- Meningiomas
- Gliomas.

Meningiomas (which compress the brain from the outside) will cause seizures, focal symptoms, and/or progressive impairment of intellectual function before they will produce a headache. The slow growth and bone invasions of these lesions probably counter the effects of their proximity to pain-sensitive structures.

Gliomas and large infiltrating tumors can advance throughout one hemisphere without causing headache because the position of the large vessels is not disturbed. These lesions may cause headache early due to their rapid growth and possible occlusion of the lateral, third and fourth ventricle.

Hematomas

The headache associated with hematomas is similar to that described previously in this chapter. There are no characteristic symptoms that will help the physician differentiate an acute subdural hematoma from a cerebral contusion or laceration. Chronic subdural hematomas may occur after trivial or closed-head trauma. Although headache is a prominent symptom of subdural hematoma, the diagnosis will be difficult to establish if the patient presents in a confused state. Other symptoms of acute subdural hematoma are:

- Drowsiness
- Confusion
- Slowness in thinking
- Occasional agitation.

These symptoms will progressively intensify. Focal and lateralizing signs occur late and are less prominent than the disturbance in consciousness. In both the subacute and chronic types of subdural hematomas, the clinical picture resembles the presentation of progressive supratentorial mass. Its characteristics include:

- Hemiparesis
- Focal seizures
- Choked discs.

In distinguishing the types of subdural hematomas, the following should be considered:

- Acute subdural hematomas usually become clinically significant within 48 hours of injury.
- Subacute subdural hematomas will become clinically significant within 2 to 14 days after injury.
- Chronic subdural hematomas will become clinically significant 14 or more days after injury.

Headache is not an important clinical sign in acute subdural hematoma since the patient is often unconscious upon admission after severe head injury. Headache may or may not be present in patients with subacute subdural hematomas. Surgical intervention is usually indicated in these patients as these hematomas rarely absorb spontaneously.

Headache is the most common complaint of patients with the chronic form. The injury experienced by these patients is usually mild to moderate, and a history of injury may be absent. If the headache is not treated, progressive signs of brain compression may occur and are often nonlocalizing and nonspecific. These symptoms include:

- Apathy
- Inappropriate behavior
- Confusion.

Sudden head movements or jolts can exacerbate the headache. Head tapping can be used as a clinical sign. In the elderly, chronic subdural hematoma may present as mental deterioration without headache.

Epidural hematoma most often presents in the patient after injury to the middle meningeal artery on the under surface of the temporal bone. As the injured patient progresses from a complaint of headache to restlessness, the physician should be concerned about the possibility of expanding intracranial mass. As the lesion increases in size and produces brain compression and decreasing levels of consciousness, the patient may be combative, restless and not necessarily complain of headache.

Subarachnoid Hemorrhage

After head injury, bleeding into the subarachnoid space may occur. It is the most common cause of intracranial hemorrhage or may be secondary to intracerebral hemorrhage. The bleeding may also occur spontaneously from:

- Preexisting aneurysms
- Vascular malformations

Rarely:
- Blood dyscrasia
- Intracranial tumor
- Some form of arteritis.

The clinical presentation for all subarachnoid hemorrhage is:
- Acute onset of severe headache
- Frontal or diffuse pain radiating to the neck, back and even the lower extremities
- The patient will describe the pain as "the worst headache ever"
- Within minutes, a variable degree of mental confusion may occur.

Blood in the subarachnoid space causes a chemical meningitis. The "meningeal signs" include:
- Stiff neck
- Kernig's sign (inability to extend the leg with the thigh flexed)
- Mildly elevated temperature, pulse and blood pressure.

Signs and symptoms following a subarachnoid hemorrhage are largely due to vascular spasm resulting in brain ischemia, infarct and cerebral edema. The cause of a subarachnoid hemorrhage may be suggested by:
- A history of progressive neurological deficits
- A history of seizure disorder
- Auscultating a cranial bruit.

These signs would suggest an intracranial vascular malformation. Aneurysms may be symptomatic before hemorrhage and cause varied degrees of headache or extraocular paresis by compression of the third cranial nerve. Easy bruising or prolonged bleeding from lumbar or venipuncture sites may indicate blood dyscrasia.

Generally, an unruptured aneurysm does not require surgical intervention. The performance of invasive diagnostic procedures should be minimized with unruptured aneurysms.

Brain Abscess

The signs and symptoms of brain abscess are comparable to those with an intracranial expanding lesion. Cerebral edema is significant in the pathophysiology. Early symptoms include:

- Headache
- Nausea
- Vomiting
- Seizures.

Brain abscess may be due to:

- Active or acute bacterial infections involving extracranial sites
- Extracranial fungal and parasitic infections.

Early diagnosis can expedite treatment measures and be established by specific procedures, including:

- Chest x-ray to rule out lung abscess
- EEG to rule out characteristic focal high-voltage waves
- Complete blood count
- Computed tomography (CT) scan or magnetic resonance imaging (MRI).

Parenchymal abscess is often associated with disease of adjacent nasal and aural structures, and the patient may experience headache from the latter source before brain tissue is actually involved. A headache will not occur until the abscess is of adequate size to cause traction and displacement, usually 2 months after the parenchymal breakdown has started. The abscess will then be of maximal size, walled off, and have become a cystic tumor that gradually developed in size from accumulation of fluid. The headache of brain abscess is usually associated with:

- Leukocytosis
- Fever
- Pleocytosis.

Brain abscess from ear infections may occur either above or below the tentorium. Evidence of brain stem embarrassment occurs early in the illness and includes:

- Hiccoughing
- Vomiting
- Occipital headache.

Epidural abscess is often present in headache associated with sinus disease and osteomyelitis of the adjacent bony wall, and which persists after drainage of the sinus. These epidural abscesses occur in the frontal region adjacent to the diseased sinus, which may be:

- Frontal sinus
- Ethmoid sinus
- Sphenoid sinus.

Also, the abscess may occur after osteomyelitis of the mastoid bone in the postauricular occipital region.

Arteriovenous Malformations

Arteriovenous malformations (AVMs) vary in size from a mass of tortuous vessels occupying most of one cerebral hemisphere to barely visible blemishes involving any part of the brain. Although an AVM may be present at birth, the symptoms may not manifest until adolescence or in early adulthood. Occasionally, the symptoms may never occur. The AVMs attain clinical significance depending on the major neurological complications associated with or caused by the malformation, including:

- Subarachnoid hemorrhage
- Seizure disorder
- Progressive neurological deficits.

The presence of AVMs can be established by CT scanning or MRI.

Infections

Headache associated with fever and stiff neck should always alert the physician to the possibility of meningitis. Meningitis may be caused by a variety of sources:

- Viral infection
- Bacterial infection
- Fungal infection
- Blood disorder
- Metastatic disease to the meninges, such as lymphoma.

The symptoms of meningitis are determined by:

- Type of structure involved
- Degree of inflammation
- Location of the inflammatory process.

The headache associated with meningitis is:

- Severe and global
- Throbbing in nature
- Associated with:
  - Nausea
  - Vomiting
  - Photophobia
  - Stiff neck
  - An alteration in the level of consciousness (occasionally)
  - Occasional occurrence of a rash.

It may be due to the extreme reflex spasm of the cervical musculature. In the early stages, with mild to moderate headache and minimal neck stiffness, the cause may be attributed to influenza. Lumbar puncture will establish the diagnosis. A morbid outcome of this disorder may be prevented with:

- Early diagnosis
- Aggressive antibiotic therapy.

Four other conditions may be mistaken for meningitis. The common element in these disorders is severe headache and/or the presence of resistance to anterior flexion of the neck. These conditions include:

- Retropharyngeal abscess, particularly in children
- Superior longitudinal sinus thrombosis
- Subarachnoid hemorrhage
- Meningismus that may accompany certain infections, such as typhoid fever.

Low Cerebrospinal Fluid Pressure Headache

The most common form of low CSF pressure headache is the post-puncture headache. This headache may be mild or severe and occur within a few hours to several days after lumbar puncture. The headache duration varies from a few days to several weeks. One in four patients undergoing lumbar puncture will experience these headaches. The pain of these headaches is described as:

- A dull, deep ache or throbbing
- Bifrontal or suboccipital
- May be associated with moderate neck stiffness.

The most recognized characteristic of these headaches is the occurrence when the patient is erect and its disappearance when the patient is horizontal. Pain may be exacerbated with shaking the head. This headache is usually resistant to all forms of treatment except bed rest in the horizontal position and the passage of time. Its cause is attributed to the loss of CSF secondary to leakage through the dural hole.

Other causes of low CSF pressure headache have been identified:

- Primary intracranial hypotension
- CSF rhinorrhea
- Inappropriate ventricular shunt.

The appropriate therapy for these disorders is correction of the cause.

Chronic or Marked Increases in Intracranial Pressure

Two disorders are identified as causing these headaches:

- Acute hydrocephalus
- Benign intracranial hypertension.

Acute hydrocephalus occurs in patients with ventricular obstruction or with shunt malfunction in a treated hydrocephalic patient. The severe headache is followed by visual disturbances. Emergency ventricular drainage must be completed rapidly to prevent permanent neurological deficit or death.

No specific cause can be established for benign intracranial hypertension (BIH) although there is evidence of increased intracranial pressure. Because this disorder can stop spontaneously, it is described as benign. However, permanent visual loss may occur. Etiological factors which may be involved include:

- Menstrual dysfunction
- Adrenal deficiency

- Corticosteroid therapy
- Hypoparathyroidism
- Vitamin A intoxication
- Tetracycline administration in infants
- Poisons
- Insecticides.

The one finding common to all these cases of BIH is papilledema. Other symptoms include:
- Generalized headache
- Giddiness
- Vomiting
- Blurred vision in some cases
- Rarely, seizures
- Patient's feeling and appearance of well-being are striking.

Pseudotumor is one of the syndromes associated with BIH. The symptoms include:
- Nonspecific, intermittent headache
- Present for several weeks or months before seeking medical advice.

There is a high incidence of this disorder in young, obese females. The resting spinal pressures vary from 220 mg to 600 mm of water. The spinal fluid is always:
- Clear
- Colorless
- Exhibiting no abnormality of cellular or chemical constituents
- Protein count of the CSF is unusually low.

Most patients respond well to acetazolamide. Some patients will require shunt placement.

Cranial Arteritis

Headaches due to cranial arteritis are related to inflammatory processes of undetermined cause, which are limited to the cranial arteries. In the process, the elasticity of the arterial walls seems to fade as the tissues appear frayed or fragmented. Giant cells within the vessel walls are most numerous in the region of the deranged internal elastic lamina. The pain is evoked by inflammatory responses that include those of the pain-sensitive structures of the head. The headaches occur coincidentally with the inflammatory process and once the disease is managed, the headaches do not recur.

Giant cell arteritis is also referred to as temporal arteritis. The classification committee of the International Headache Society requires one of the following criteria to establish the diagnosis of giant cell arteritis:

- Swollen and tender scalp artery (usually superficial temporal artery)
- Elevated RBC sedimentation rate
- Disappearance of headache within 48 hours of the initiation of steroid therapy.

Diagnosis is confirmed with a temporal artery biopsy that will demonstrate giant cell arteritis.

The physician should be alert to this disorder in patients over age 50 experiencing recent onset of headache. The physician should obtain a sedimentation rate by Westergren's method on all patients over age 50. In patients with giant cell arteritis, the sedimentation rate is usually above 60 mm/hr, although some patients may present with normal sedimentation rates. Early diagnosis and treatment are essential to prevent the irreversible blindness associated with this disorder.

The headache is probably the most prominent presenting complaint. Patients will describe it as:

- Very severe intensity
- Often unilateral, localized over one temple; however, the pain may be bilateral
- Throbbing or boring
- Occasionally, a stabbing sensation across the temporal area
- Often having a burning component.

The headache is often worse when the patient lies flat in bed and decreases in severity when the patient is sitting upright. Applying pressure to the common carotid artery may diminish the pain, and stooping may exacerbate the pain.

Many patients will present a history similar to rheumatoid arthritis and giant cell arteritis is often associated with polymyalgia rheumatica. Other symptoms include:

- Night sweating
- Aching of the joints
- Fever
- Weight loss.

The patient may experience pain or discomfort on opening the mouth as well as pain and stiffness in the area of the temporomandibular joint. Intermittent claudication of the jaw may be triggered by excessive chewing, thus resulting in weight loss. Facial swelling and red nodules may be observed over the temporal region. The visual symptoms may develop 5 or more months after the symptoms manifest. These symptoms are believed to be caused by a decrease in the blood supply to the optic nerve, and include:

- Ophthalmoplegia
- Diplopia
- Ptosis
- Other symptoms of ocular motor paralysis.

Resultant ischemia of the optic nerve occurs in about 50% of untreated patients. Many patients with untreated giant cell arteritis may experience transient visual blurring before the onset of the irreversible blindness.

Because imminent treatment is essential to prevent the blindness, therapy with corticosteroids should be initiated before receiving the results of the biopsy. The usual starting dose is prednisone 40 mg to 60 mg daily. Maintenance dose is 10 mg to 20 mg per day, with the sedimentation rate used as a guide in administering the drug. The disease process usually disappears 6 to 8 months after initiation of therapy.

Before the major manifestation of giant cell arteritis, pain may occur in other areas including:

- Teeth
- Jaw
- Ear
- Zygoma
- Nuchal area
- Occiput.

These symptoms indicate involvement of other branches of the external carotid artery, particularly the external and internal maxillary arteries. Other arteries may be involved including:

- Major vessels of the aorta
- Coronary arteries
- Arteries of the limbs.

The large and medium size arteries are the principal sites of the inflammatory process.

Major Neuralgias

Major neuralgias include trigeminal neuralgia and glossopharyngeal neuralgia. Trigeminal neuralgia is also known as tic douloureux. Characteristically, trigeminal neuralgia consists of:

- Episodic, recurrent pain
- Unilateral location, more common on the right side of the face
- Rarely begins before age 50
- Female to male ratio is 2:1.

This disorder rarely occurs before age 30 unless the patient has concomitant multiple sclerosis.

The pain is of high intensity and particularly affects trigger zones that are increased areas of sensitivity on the face, especially above the nares and mouth. When stimulated, these areas will trigger the attacks, often by trivial stimulation. Because of these trigger zones, the patient will demonstrate the "avoidance mechanism." This mechanism is a major diagnostic clue. The patient with trigeminal neuralgia will typically avoid washing the face, shaving, chewing or any other action that will stimulate a trigger zone. Because many trigger zones are located in or near the oral cavity, patients with trigeminal neuralgia will lose a great deal of weight.

The distribution of trigeminal neuralgia affects the second or third divisions of the fifth cranial nerve and will radiate to the first division late in the disease. Patients have described the pain as:

- Short, sharp, momentary bursts, like electric shock or a rapid repeating rifle
- Excruciating and severe enough to cause the patient to cry out or twitch
- Periods of remission are interrupted by attacks caused by stimulation of the trigger zones
- High intensity jabs last less than 20 to 30 seconds with short-term remission periods lasting a few seconds, followed by another jab of pain.

Treatment of choice for trigeminal neuralgia is anticonvulsant therapy. These drugs will reduce the sensitivity of the trigger zones as well as relieve the pain, often dramatically, within hours after initiation of therapy. Table 3.1 reviews the agents used for trigeminal neuralgia. Initial therapy is carbamazepine 100 mg to 200 mg 2 or 3 times per day. If this dose is well tolerated and if the pain is quickly relieved, the drug may be continued for an indefinite period, depending on the course of the disease. Severity of the pain will determine the titration of the drug. Maintenance dose is usually 200 mg per day.

TABLE 3.1 — PHARMACOLOGIC TREATMENT OF TRIGEMINAL NEURALGIA		
Generic (Trade) Name	Dose	Side Effects
Carbamazepine (Tegretol)	200-600 mg	Blood disorders
Phenytoin (Dilantin)	200-400 mg	CNS symptoms, hemopoietic, oral
Chlorphenesin (Maolate)	800-2400 mg	Drowsiness
Baclofen (Lioresal)	30-80 mg	Drowsiness, weakness, nausea, vomiting
Abbreviations: CNS, central nervous system.		

If the symptoms persist, phenytoin may be added to the regimen in doses up to 400 mg per day. Chlorphenesin should be considered if the patient is refractory to the first two agents. This drug is prescribed in doses of 400 mg 3 to 4 times daily. Surgical intervention may be considered if the patient has reached a three-drug treatment level. Baclofen has been used successfully in refractory trigeminal neuralgia at doses of 60 mg to 80 mg per day.

The final stage in therapy may be surgical intervention (Table 3.2). Surgical procedures should only be considered after other methods have failed and include:

- Glycerol injections
- Radiofrequency rhizotomy
- Microsurgical decompression of the trigeminal root.

TABLE 3.2 — SURGICAL PROCEDURES FOR TRIGEMINAL NEURALGIA		
Procedure	**Benefits**	**Contraindications**
Glycerol injection	• 85% effective • No craniotomy • Minor procedure	• Masseter weakness • Facial sensory loss
Radiofrequency rhizotomy	• 90% effective • Minor procedure • Brief hospitalization	• Facial sensory loss • Facial weakness • Corneal hypesthesia (10% to 15%)
Microvascular decompression of the trigeminal root	• 90% effective • No sensory loss	• Major craniotomy • ± 4% critical postoperative complications • 1% mortality • Prolonged hospitalization

Because the decompression of the trigeminal root requires a formal craniotomy, resulting in extended hospitalizations and convalescence, glycerol injections are preferred. These injections are accomplished rapidly.

Glossopharyngeal neuralgia is similar to trigeminal neuralgia except that the symptoms manifest from the anatomical base of the glossopharyngeal nerve. This pain is usually located in the:

- Pharynx
- Tonsils
- Ear.

It can be triggered by swallowing, yawning or eating. Treatment is similar to that of trigeminal neuralgia.

Certain atypical neuralgias may present which cannot be categorized according to the symptomatology and are not associated with trigger zones. The pain does not occur as jabs but rather as continuous pain. Atypical facial pain can be described as:

- Steady diffuse aching, not neuritic
- Continuous for hours, days, months
- No trigger zones
- Often localized tenderness
- May have a vascular component
- May radiate to other regions of the face, neck, cranium.

Autonomic symptoms may also occur and include:

- Cutaneous pallor
- Sweating
- Flushing
- Rhinitis.

To alter the responses to autonomic stimuli, the patient may respond to β-blockers, including propranolol. Due to the chronic nature of atypical facial pain, the patient has the potential to develop depression or habituation problems. A multidisciplinary approach to this patient, possibly in an inpatient facility, may be indicated. Psychological testing and counseling may be required in patients with atypical facial pain. Treatment measures include:

- Non-habituating analgesics
- Antidepressants
- Nerve blocks
- Transcutaneous electrical stimulation
- Biofeedback
- Psychological counseling.

Some patients will experience postinfectious neuralgia, particularly as a complication of herpes zoster of the face and head. This neuralgia most often affects the elderly. Most of these affected patients will demonstrate pain with involvement of the gasserian ganglion. In some patients, the ophthalmic division of the nerve is infected, or present with a herpetic rash in the external auditory canal with facial palsy (Ramsay Hunt syndrome). Unfortunately, the pain of postherpetic neuralgia will dominate the remaining years of these patients. The pain of postherpetic neuralgia has been described as:

- Steady and sustained
- Almost always unilateral
- Burning and aching
- Frequently interrupts sleep.

Diagnosis is usually obvious as the scars of the herpetic eruption are apparent, and trophic changes to the skin may result from this disorder. The pain of herpes zoster usually abates within 2 to 3 weeks although the neuralgia may persist for months or years.

These patients also tend to develop depression and dependency problems. The tricyclic antidepressants may be beneficial although the dose increases should be undertaken cautiously in elderly patients. The addition of a phenothiazine may be considered. These patients require reassurance and patience, and may need psychological counseling. Surgical intervention is not indicated for these patients.

Temporomandibular Joint Disorder

Temporomandibular joint (TMJ) disorder is one of the most overly publicized and overly diagnosed disorders. Symptoms of TMJ disorder include:

- Localized facial pain
- Limitation of motion of the jaw

- Muscle tenderness
- Joint crepitus.

The pain of TMJ disorder is usually localized in front of and behind the ear on the affected side. This pain may radiate over the cheek and face. X-rays of the jaw are usually normal. Due to the localized pain, the patient will always use the opposite side of the mouth for chewing, thus splinting the painful side. There is no evidence that hearing loss, damage to the cranial nerves, disturbances of equilibrium, development of Ménière's syndrome, or difficulty with the eustachian tubes are associated with TMJ disorder.

Pain relief of TMJ disorder should be directed toward abating muscle spasm. Mouth reconstructions are usually not indicated and extensive oral surgery should not be undertaken unless other measures have failed. Simple analgesics and muscle relaxant agents, such as chlorphenesin, may be beneficial. Non-drug methods, such as heat, hot packs and massage, may be beneficial. Dental splints and similar procedures may prove helpful.

REFERENCES

AbuRahma AF, Thaxton L. Temporal arteritis: diagnostic and therapeutic considerations. *Am Surg*. 1996;62:449-451.

Dalessio DJ. The major neuralgias, postinfectious neuritis, and atypical facial pain. In: Dalessio DJ, Silberstein SD, (eds). *Wolff's Headache and Other Head Pain*, 6th ed. New York, NY: Oxford University Press; 1993:345-364.

Diamond S. Head pain. Diagnosis and management. *Clin Symp*. 1994;46:2-34.

Francis JH, Pennal BE, Hold CR. Medical-dental headache treatment controversy. *Headache Q*. 1995;6:208-211.

Jaeckle KA. Causes and management of headaches in cancer patients. *Oncology*. 1993;7:27-31.

Jakobsson KE. Síaveland H, Hillman J, et al. Warning leak and management outcome in aneurysmal subarachnoid hemorrhage. *J Neurosurg*. 1996;85:995-999.

Kupersmith MJ, Vargas ME, Yashar A, et al. Occipital arteriovenous malformations: visual disturbances and presentation. *Neurology*. 1996;46:953-957.

Mathew NT, Ravishankar K, Sanin LC. Coexistence of migraine and idiopathic intracranial hypertension without papilledema. *Neurology*. 1996;46:1226-1230.

McConaha C, Bastiani AM, Kaye WH. Significant reduction of post-lumbar puncture headaches by the use of a 29-gauge spinal needle. *Biol Psychiatry*. 1996;39:1058-1060.

Melo TP, Pinto AN, Ferro JM. Headache in intracerebral hematomas. *Neurology*. 1996;47:494-500.

Nathan PE, Sonenblick D, Chakote V, Wolf R, Sacchi TJ. Headache, thrombolytic therapy, and chronic subdural hemorrhage – a case report. *Angiology*. 1994;45:77-80.

Neal JM. Postdural puncture headache: prevention and treatment. *Prog Anesthesiol*. 1994;8:223-233.

Silberstein SD, Marcelis J. Headache associated with changes in intracranial pressure. *Headache*. 1992;32:84-94.

Storrs TJ, Roberts CI. Adult Chiari malformation with headache and trigeminal dysesthesia. *Oral Surg Oral Med Oral Pathol Oral Radiol Endod*. 1996;82:284-287.

van den Bergh R, van Calenbergh F. Headache and headache attacks in the Chiari-I malformation and in syringomyelia. *Headache Q*. 1997;8:15-21.

Verma A, Rosenfeld V, Forteza A, Sharma KR. Occipital lobe tumor presenting as migraine with typical aura. *Headache*. 1996;36:49-52.

4   Migraine Headaches

Migraine is defined by the Classification Committee of the International Headache Society (IHS) as: Idiopathic, recurring headache disorder manifesting in attacks lasting 4 to 72 hours. Typical characteristics of headache are:

- Unilateral location
- Pulsating quality
- Moderate or severe intensity
- Aggravation by routine physical activity
- Association with nausea
- Photo- and phonophobia.

Diagnosis

The distinctive feature of migraine with aura is the complex of focal neurological symptoms, which gradually develop over 5 to 20 minutes and usually last less than 60 minutes. These symptoms usually occur 30 to 60 minutes before the onset of an acute migraine attack. Symptoms include:

- Diagnostic features
- Clinical features.

■ Diagnostic Features

Up to 70% of migraine sufferers have a positive family history of migraine headaches. There is a preponderance in migraine with approximately 70% of migraine sufferers being female.

Onset of migraine usually starts during adolescence and the early twenties. Migraine tends to diminish in the fifth and sixth decades.

Headache triggers include:
- Stress
- Fatigue
- Oversleeping
- Fasting or missing a meal
- Vasoactive substances in foods
- Caffeine
- Alcohol
- Menses
- Changes in barometric pressure
- Changes in altitude.

Medications that may precipitate migraine include:
- Reserpine
- Nitrates
- Indomethacin
- Oral contraceptives
- Post-menopausal hormones.

Personality features of migraine patients are a topic of debate and include perfectionism, rigidity and compulsiveness. Migraine patients tend to build environments too great to handle.

■ Clinical Features

Migraines are usually unilateral headaches but may occur bilaterally or switch sides. They are recurring headaches with a frequency of two to eight attacks per month. The duration of attack is 4 to 24 hours, although some attacks are prolonged.

Severity of pain varies from moderate to incapacitating. The pain is often described as throbbing or pulsating. Associated symptoms include:
- Nausea
- Vomiting
- Photo- and/or phonophobia
- Facial pallor
- Vertigo

- Tinnitus
- Irritability.

Prodrome symptoms associated with migraine with aura include (in order of frequency):
- Scotomata (blind spots)
- Teichopsia (fortification spectrum)
- Photopsia (flashing of lights)
- Visual and auditory hallucinations.

Premonitory symptoms may precede an attack of migraine with or without aura. These symptoms include:
- Bursts of energy
- Fatigue
- Extreme hunger
- Nervousness.

Types of Migraine

Types of migraine include:
- Migraine with aura
- Migraine without aura
- Complicated migraine
- Menstrual migraine
- Migraine equivalents.

Complicated migraine consists of acute attacks which may be accompanied by neurological symptoms which may persist after headache has subsided. These types include:
- Hemiplegic migraine
- Ophthalmoplegic migraine
- Basilar migraine.

Diagnostic tests are usually negative in their findings but should be performed to rule out organic disease.

A positive family history of similar headaches is usually present.

Approximately 70% of all migraine sufferers are female, and about 70% of these female migraineurs will describe a relationship between their headaches and their menstrual periods. They will experience headaches a few days before, during and immediately after the menses. Some will relate the onset of the headaches to the menarche.

The Classification Committee of the IHS describes migraine equivalents as migraine aura without headache (this syndrome has also been termed acephalic headache). Older patients who had previously experienced migraine with aura will note that they are experiencing the prodromata without the appearance of an acute headache.

Abdominal migraine (which may occur in children) may be characterized with cyclical vomiting or periodic attacks of vertigo in normally healthy children

■ **Treatment**

Migraine treatment can be divided into four types:
- General treatment measures
- Abortive therapy
- Pain relief measures
- Prophylactic therapy.

General treatment measures include:
- *Maintain regular sleeping schedule*: Migraine attacks may be precipitated by fatigue or oversleeping. On weekends, holidays and during vacations, patients should awaken at the same time each day.
- *Maintain regular meal schedule*: Migraine attacks may be triggered by missing a meal or fasting. Meals should be consumed at the same time daily, and the patient should eat breakfast

at a regular time each day to avoid the week-
end or holiday headache.

- *Diet*: Migraine patients may benefit from a
  tyramine-restrictive diet and should avoid most
  foods containing vasoactive substances (Table
  4.1). Migraine sufferers should also limit intake of caffeine-containing substances.
- *Coping strategies*: Stress may be impossible to
  avoid, but the patient may learn to handle stress
  and also practice relaxation methods. The patient should learn to identify particular stressors
  and avoid these triggers. Progressive relaxation
  and breathing exercises may be of particular
  help.

■ Pharmacological Therapy

The pharmacological management of migraine
may be divided into three categories:
- Abortive
- Pain relief
- Prophylactic.

The severity, frequency and impact on the patient's
daily life will influence the type of therapy to be selected (Figure 4.1).

Abortive Therapy

For those patients with less than two headaches
per month, abortive therapy may be selected (Table
4.2) using:
- Ergotamine tartrate preparations
- Dihydroergotamine (DHE) mesylate
- Sumatriptan succinate
- Isometheptene mucate
- Combination agent of aspirin, acetaminophen
  and caffeine
- Nonsteroidal anti-inflammatory agents (NSAIDs)

TABLE 4.1 — TYRAMINE-FREE DIET

Food Item	Foods Allowed	Foods to Avoid
Beverages	Decaffeinated coffee, fruit juice, club soda, noncola soda (7-UP, gingerale). Limit caffeine sources to 2 cups/day (coffee, tea, cola).	Chocolate, cocoa, alcoholic beverages.
Meat, fish, poultry	Fresh or frozen turkey, chicken, fish, beef, lamb, veal, pork; egg as meat substitute (limit three eggs/week); tuna or tuna salad.	Aged, canned, cured or processed meat, including ham or game; pickled herring, salted dried fish; chicken livers; bologna; fermented sausage; any food prepared with meat tenderizer, soy sauce or brewer's yeast; any food containing nitrates, nitrites or tyramine.
Dairy products	Milk: homogenized, 2% or skim; cheese: American, cottage, farmer, ricotta, cream, Velveeta; yogurt (limit ½ cup/day).	Cultured dairy products (buttermilk, sour cream); chocolate milk; cheese: bleu, Boursault, brick, Brie types, Camembert types, cheddar, Gouda, mozzerella, Parmesan, provolone, romano, Roquefort, Stilton, Swiss (emmentaler).
Bread, cereal	Commercial bread, English muffins, melba toast, crackers, RyKrisp, bagel; all hot and dry cereals.	Hot, fresh, homemade yeast bread; bread or crackers containing cheese; fresh yeast coffee cake, doughnuts, sourdough bread; any product containing chocolate or nuts.
Potato or substitute	White potato, sweet potato, rice, macaroni, spaghetti, noodles.	None.

Vegetable	Any except those to avoid.	Beans such as broad, fava, garbanzo, Italian, lima, navy, pinto, pole; snow peas, pea pods; sauerkraut; onions (except for flavoring); olives; pickles.
Fruit	Any except those to avoid, limit citrus fruits to ½ cup/day, limit banana to ½ per day.	Avocados, figs, raisins, papaya, passion fruit, red plums.
Soup	Cream soups made from foods allowed in diet, homemade broths.	Canned soup, soup or bouillon cubes, soup base with autolytic yeast or MSG. (*Read labels.*)
Dessert	Fruit allowed in diet; any cake, pudding, cookies or ice cream without chocolate or nuts; JELL-O.	Chocolate ice cream, pudding, cookies, cakes or pies; mincemeat pie; nuts; any yeast-containing doughs and/or pastries.
Sweets	Sugar, jelly, jam, honey, hard candy.	Chocolate candy or syrup, carob.
Miscellaneous	Salt in moderation, lemon juice, butter or margarine, cooking oil, whipped cream, white vinegar, and commercial salad dressings in small amounts.	Pizza; cheese sauce; MSG in excessive amounts; yeast and yeast extract; meat tenderizer (Accent); seasoned salt; mixed dishes: macaroni and cheese, beef stroganoff, cheese blintzes, lasagna, frozen TV dinners; nuts: peanuts, peanut butter; seeds: pumpkin, sesame, sunflower; any pickled, preserved or marinated food. *Read labels* on snack items.

FIGURE 4.1 — TREATING MIGRAINES

(Decision points in heavy outline.)

Having diagnosed migraine, consider appropriate methods to control the patient's headaches.

General measures should be implemented, including diet, regularly scheduled meals, adequate sleep and avoiding stress.

If patient has two or more attacks per month, or the attacks are prolonged, consider prophylactic therapy in addition to abortive therapy.

If the attack is accompanied by nausea and vomiting, consider the use of antiemetics, including phenothiazines.

Prescribe abortive therapy for the acute attacks. Abortive agents to be considered include:
• Ergotamine tartrate
• Dihydroergotamine

Does the patient experience another migraine during the next few days?

YES

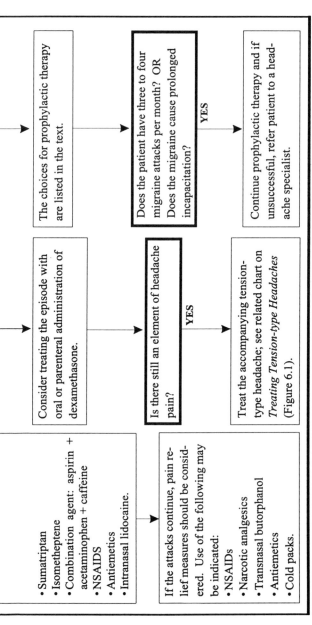

The choices for prophylactic therapy are listed in the text.

Does the patient have three to four migraine attacks per month? OR Does the migraine cause prolonged incapacitation?

YES

Continue prophylactic therapy and if unsuccessful, refer patient to a headache specialist.

Consider treating the episode with oral or parenteral administration of dexamethasone.

Is there still an element of headache pain?

YES

Treat the accompanying tension-type headache; see related chart on *Treating Tension-type Headaches* (Figure 6.1).

• Sumatriptan
• Isometheptene
• Combination agent: aspirin + acetaminophen + caffeine
• NSAIDS
• Antiemetics
• Intranasal lidocaine.

If the attacks continue, pain relief measures should be considered. Use of the following may be indicated:
• NSAIDs
• Narcotic analgesics
• Transnasal butorphanol
• Antiemetics
• Cold packs.

TABLE 4.2 — MIGRAINE ABORTIVE THERAPY

Generic Name	Trade Name	Route	Dosage
Ergotamine tartrate with caffeine	Cafergot Wigraine	Oral	Two tablets immediately at onset, may repeat every $1/2$ hour, up to six tablets/day, 10 tablets/week.
	Cafergot	Rectal	Insert one suppository immediately at onset, may repeat in 1 hour, up to two suppositories/day, five/week.
Dihydroergotamine	D.H.E. 45	Intramuscular, subcutaneous	1 mg at onset, may repeat at hourly intervals, up to three injections/day.
	Migranal	Intranasal	2 mg, one spray in each nostril; repeat in 15 minutes, up to 3 mg/day.
Sumatriptan	Imitrex	Subcutaneous	6 mg at onset, may repeat dose in 1 hour, up to 12 mg/day.
		Oral	Start with 25-50 mg at onset. If ineffective, dose can be repeated in 2 hours, up to 100 mg.
		Intranasal	20 mg, one spray in one nostril at onset, may repeat within 2 to 24 hours, limited to two sprays/day.

Isometheptene mucate with dichloralphenazone and acetaminophen	Midrin	Oral	Two capsules at onset, may be repeated every hour, up to five capsules/day, 15/week.
Aspirin, acetaminophen and caffeine	Extra-Strength Excedrin	Oral	Two tablets at onset, may repeat in 4 hours. If headache persists, professional help should be sought.
Naproxen sodium	Anaprox	Oral	825 mg initially, and 550 mg after 1 hour.
Ketorolac	Toradol	Intramuscular	60 mg at onset.
Chlorpromazine	Thorazine	Intramuscular	50-100 mg
Prochlorperazine	Compazine	Intramuscular	10-25 mg
Lidocaine	—	Intranasal	15 drops of 4% solution to the nostril ipsilateral to the pain. May be repeated in 5 minutes, up to 4 times/day.

- Phenothiazines
- Intranasal lidocaine.

During the past three decades, research has suggested a relationship between serotonin (5-HT) and migraine. One theory portends that migraine attacks are triggered by the release of 5-HT from the platelets. Another theory indicates that the release of 5-HT from perivascular terminals of putative serotonergic nerve fibers initiates the acute attack. Another precipitating event has been suggested – systemic metabolic changes in 5-HT metabolism. It is known that serotonergic drugs, such as reserpine, can provoke a migraine attack. Sterile neurogenic inflammation has been suggested as the cause of migraine pain. Stimulation of the trigeminal ganglion in the rat results in the release of substance P and calcitonin- generated peptide which produces neurogenic plasma extravasation, an event which can be blocked by the $5\text{-}HT_1$ agonists.

Agents recognized as 5-HT agonists, such as ergotamine, DHE, and sumatriptan, have demonstrated efficacy in aborting migraine attacks and have variable affinity for the $5\text{-}HT_{1A}$, $5\text{-}HT_{1B}$, $5\text{-}HT_{1D}$, and $5\text{-}HT_{1F}$ receptors. Their anti-migraine effect is exerted by a receptor-mediated neural pathway in both the central nervous system and in the trigeminal nerve, where they block neurogenic inflammation.

Repeated daily doses over an extended interval of any of these 5-HT receptor agonists may cause a rebound phenomena. This should be distinguished by the clinician from a headache reoccurrence which may present from 2 to 12 hours after one dose of the agent.

Ergotamine Tartrate Preparations

Ergotamine tartrate preparations are vasoconstrictors that have been used in migraine abortive therapy for over 50 years. These agents are available for oral (Cafergot, Wigraine) and rectal (Cafergot) administration in combination with caffeine. Ergotamine is also available for sublingual administration (Ergostat). It is no longer available in the United States in the parenteral form. An adequate dose should be taken as early as possible in the attack to achieve a maximum response.

To prevent ergotamine rebound headaches or ergotism, care should be taken to remain within the limits of recommended dosage. Ergotamine tartrate should not be used in patients with:

- Cerebrovascular disease
- Cardiovascular disease
- Peripheral vascular disease
- Severe hypertension
- Ischemic heart disease
- Sepsis
- Renal disease
- Hepatic disease.

Ergotamine should be used cautiously in patients with:
- Peptic ulcer
- Recent infection.

Ergotamine should not be used in pregnancy.

Dihydroergotamine Mesylate

Dihydroergotamine mesylate (D.H.E. 45) has also been used safely and effectively in the abortive therapy of migraine for over 50 years, but it has recently been "rediscovered" as a $5-HT_1$ receptor agonist. In addition to the $5-HT_{1D}$ receptor, DHE is also potent at a number of other biogenic amine receptors. Unlike ergotamine tartrate, DHE is associated with less nausea and is more of a venoconstrictor than an arterial vasoconstrictor. DHE can also be used to help "detox" patients who are ergotamine dependent.

Dihydroergotamine is available in 1 mg/mL ampules for parenteral administration (IM, SC, IV). Onset of action occurs within 15 to 30 minutes after IM injection, and continues for 3 to 4 hours. When given IM or SC, 70% to 77% of the patients obtained relief. Given IV, DHE produces less nausea than ergotamine. In patients with intractable migraine, DHE given in repetitive IV doses has been successful. DHE 0.5 mg given IV push, over 2 to 3 minutes, in combination with metoclopramide (Reglan) 10 mg may be repeated every 8 hours for 3 days to treat intractable migraine.

The route of administration is important in obtaining relief because it impacts on the speed of action. Although oral administration is the most simple route, it may not be indicated in the 70% of migraineurs who experience associated nausea and vomiting. Also, the oral preparation of DHE is not adequately absorbed and has low bioavailability. Parenteral administration offers the quickest action but self-injection techniques may not be the choice for many patients. Receiving an injection at a physician's office or emergency department may delay the quick action so badly needed.

Recently, a more acceptable form of administration, intranasal, has been approved. The efficacy of the 2 mg dose was demonstrated in two recent studies comparing intranasal DHE (Migranal) versus placebo. For those patients using oral preparations of 5-HT receptor agonists and requiring increasing doses or who are considered treatment failures to the 5-HT receptor agonists, DHE nasal spray may be a viable alternative. Headache recurrence rates are low, observed in only 14% of patients after the use of DHE nasal spray. The low recurrence rate seen with DHE may be due to its tight binding to the 5-HT receptor and slow drug-receptor dissociation.

Due to its vasoconstrictive properties, DHE is contraindicated in patients with:

- Peripheral arterial disease
- Ischemic heart disease
- Prinzmetal's angina
- Uncontrolled hypertension
- Hemiplegic or basilar migraine
- Impaired hepatic or renal function
- Sepsis
- Pregnancy
- Hypersensitivity to ergot alkaloids.

DHE should not be used concomitantly with $5\text{-}HT_1$ agonists (sumatriptan) or ergotamine preparations.

It is recommended that DHE not be given to patients in whom unrecognized coronary artery disease (CAD) is predicted by the presence of risk factors unless a cardiovascular evaluation provides satisfactory clinical evidence that a patient is reasonably free of CAD, ischemic myocardial disease, or other significant underlying cardiovascular disease.

For patients with risk factors predictive of CAD who have a satisfactory cardiovascular evaluation, it is recommended that the initial dose be administered in a physician's office, unless the patient has previously received DHE. Because cardiac ischemia can occur in the absence of clinical symptoms, consideration should be given to obtaining, on the first use, an electrocardiogram (EKG) during the interval following administration in patients with risk factors.

Triptans

Sumatriptan (Imitrex) is a novel selective agent of 5-hydroxytryptamine (5-HT)-like receptors, which are believed to be membranal "trigger" proteins with which 5-HT must interact to produce its various actions. These actions include dilation of certain cranial arteries or arteriovenous anastomoses by neurogenic dural plasma extravasation, or both mechanisms which in turn will trigger a migraine. Sumatriptan blocks these phenomena and has demonstrated efficacy in migraine abortive therapy.

During migraine attacks, an oral dose of sumatriptan 100 mg provides improvement within 2 hours in 56% of patients and within 4 hours in approximately 75% of patients. Seventy percent to 80% of patients report improvement within 1 hour after SC injection of 6 mg. Alternative routes of administration have also been investigated for sumatriptan. The intranasal administration of this agent, in a 20 mg dose, has demonstrated efficacy in 61% of patients at 120 minutes after use.

Since sumatriptan became available in 1991, several reports have been generated on clinical experience. In studies comparing it to placebo, side effects were most often brief and mild to moderate in intensity, and included:
- Tingling sensation
- Constriction of throat
- Chest pain and pressure
- Heaviness in limbs.

Limitations of sumatriptan use include the presentation of chest symptoms, which may or may not indicate cardiac ischemia due to vasoconstriction of coronary arteries, recurrence of the headache within 24 hours after initial successful treatment of an attack, and in a few patients, abuse of the agent possibly due to rebound phenomena.

Because of its potential to cause coronary vasospasms, sumatriptan should never be administered by IV. In addition, it should not be used concomitantly with ergotamine preparations or monoamine oxidase inhibitors (MAOIs).

Sumatriptan is contraindicated in patients with:

- Ischemic heart disease (or presenting with symptoms or signs consistent with ischemic heart disease)
- Prizmetal's angina
- Uncontrolled hypertension
- Hemiplegic or basilar migraine
- Pregnancy
- Hypersensitivity to sumatriptan.

It is recommended that sumatriptan not be given to patients in whom unrecognized coronary artery disease is predicted by the presence of risk factors for CAD, unless a cardiovascular evaluation provides satisfactory clinical evidence that the patient is reasonably free of coronary artery and ischemic myocardial disease or other significant underlying cardiovascular disease.

For patients with risk factors predictive of CAD who have a satisfactory cardiovascular evaluation, it is recommended that the initial dose be administered in a physician's office. Because cardiac ischemia can occur in the absence of clinical symptoms, consideration should be given to obtaining, on the first use, an EKG during the interval following administration in patients with risk factors.

Three new oral triptan agents, naratriptan (Amerge), zolmitriptan (Zomig), and rizatriptan (Maxalt) are expected to be available by the end of 1998 in the United States. Naratriptan is a second generation 5-HT_{1D} receptor agonist, and zolmitriptan and rizatriptan are selective $5\text{-HT}_{1D/1B}$ receptor agonists. The advantages or disadvantages of these newer agents will be judged on their clinical experience.

Isometheptene Mucate

In patients who cannot tolerate ergotamine or in whom these drugs are contraindicated, isometheptene mucate may be effective. Similar to ergotamine, iso-metheptene has cerebral vasoconstrictive actions. Isometheptene is available in a preparation with dichloralphenazone and acetaminophen (Midrin).

Aspirin, Acetaminophen and Caffeine

The most recently approved agent to the list of migraine abortives is a combination of aspirin, acetaminophen and caffeine (Extra-Strength Excedrin). It is the first over-the-counter (OTC) preparation to receive approval for this indication. This combination agent is suggested for the acute treatment of mild-to-moderate headache without associated vomiting and disability.

Nonsteroidal Anti-inflammatory Agents

The NSAIDs in migraine abortive therapy have been used successfully with several of these agents. The NSAIDS stabilize proteins and inhibit the formation of active prostaglandins from their precursors. NSAIDs inhibit inflammation through their effects on:
- Chemotaxis
- Phagocytosis
- Lysosomal enzyme release
- Kinin generation.

NSAIDS available include:
- Naproxen sodium (Anaprox, Aleve)
- Ibuprofen
- Aspirin.

A parenteral form of the NSAIDs is available. Ketorolac (Toradol) is advantageous as it offers a parenteral analgesic which:
- Is non-narcotic
- Is non-habituating
- Has a low side effect profile.

Ketorolac is administered in doses of 60 mg IM.

Phenothiazines

The phenothiazines have been used effectively in the emergency department setting for the abortive treatment of acute migraine. Their efficacy is attributed to their antinauseant and sedative effects. In addition, their dopaminergic and adrenergic actions may provide specific mechanisms for aborting migraine. The phenothiazines used in migraine abortive therapy include:
- Chlorpromazine (Thorazine)
- Prochlorperazine (Compazine).

Intranasal Lidocaine

A recent report has suggested the use of intranasal lidocaine as a viable agent for the abortive treatment of an acute migraine attack. A 50% reduction in headache was noted by 55% of patients treated with lidocaine. Relapse was common and occurred early after treatment. In this author's clinical experience, this treatment has particularly demonstrated significant benefit.

Pain Relief

Complete resolution of the attack may not be achieved by abortive therapy and analgesics may be indicated. These agents include OTC analgesics:
- Aspirin
- Acetaminophen
- Ibuprofen
- Naproxen sodium
- Ketoprofen (Orudis).

Overconsumption of these analgesics, particularly OTC analgesics containing caffeine, can produce serious side effects. Withdrawal from caffeine-containing drugs may trigger the caffeine withdrawal headache. These drugs should be avoided in those patients with frequent migraine attacks.

Other pain-relief measures for the acute migraine attacks include:

- Narcotic analgesics
- Antiemetics
- Transnasal butorphanol
- Cold packs.

Narcotic Analgesics

The use of the narcotic analgesics, preferably administered parenterally, is acknowledged effective for pain relief. As with other pain syndromes, these drugs should not be used in patients with frequently occurring migraine attacks. Narcotic analgesics used in relief of acute attacks include:

- Codeine
- Meperidine (Demerol)
- Methadone (Dolophine).

Antiemetics

The antiemetics are used parenterally or rectally due to the associated symptoms of nausea and vomiting. The phenothiazines are also useful for their sedative action in relieving the symptom complex present in an acute migraine attack. These drugs include:

- Promethazine (Phenergan)
- Chlorpromazine (Thorazine)
- Prochlorperazine (Compazine).

Some antiemetics have little sedative effect, including:

- Trimethobenzamide (Tigan)
- Metoclopramide (Reglan).

Metoclopramide, a 5-HT$_3$ receptor agonist, has been shown to enhance the absorption of oral medications and has been used effectively in combination with DHE IV. This drug will occasionally cause nervousness and tremor.

Transnasal Butorphanol

Transnasal butorphanol (Stadol) is a totally synthetic mixed agonist-antagonist opioid analgesic which originally was available for parenteral administration. Its quick absorption via the transnasal route is enhanced by its lipophilic nature. The highly vascular nature of the nasal mucosa renders it conducive for rapid intake and absorption of agents via the transnasal route.

Cold Packs

Cold packs have been used for many years by migraine patients. The use of ice bags or commercially manufactured ice packs, along with pressure, may reduce the pulsating pain associated with acute migraine attacks.

Prophylactic Therapy

For those patients experiencing more than two migraine attacks per month, prophylactic therapy may be considered. Prophylactic therapy is also indicated for patients complaining of attacks lasting for several days per week, or of a degree of severity that critically impacts on the patient's daily life. Several agents have been used successfully in migraine prophylaxis (Table 4.3):

- β-Blockers
- Methysergide
- Calcium channel blockers
- Neuroleptics

TABLE 4.3 — MIGRAINE PROPHYLACTIC THERAPY

Generic Name	Trade Name	Dosage
β-*Blockers*		
Propranolol	Inderal	80-240 mg daily in divided doses
	Inderal LA	60-160 mg in once daily dosing
Timolol maleate	Blocadren	5-30 mg daily
Nadolol	Corgard	40-80 mg daily
Atenolol	Tenormin	50-100 mg BID
Metoprolol	Lopressor, Toprol	50-100 mg BID
Calcium Channel Blockers		
Verapamil	Calan, Isoptin, Verelan	240-360 mg daily in divided doses
Nimodipine	Nimotop	30-60 mg daily
Alpha Agonist		
Clonidine	Catapres-TTS	0.1 mg TID
Antidepressants		
Amitriptyline	Elavil	50-100 mg Q HS
Protriptyline	Vivactil	5-10 mg TID
Phenelzine	Nardil	15 mg TID
Nonsteroidal Anti-inflammatory Agents		
Naproxen	Naprosyn, Naprelan	250 mg TID
Ketoprofen	Orudis	75 mg TID
Fenoprofen calcium	Nalfon	300 mg QID or 600 mg daily
Tolmetin sodium	Tolectin	200 mg TID
Aspirin	—	325-650 mg daily

Neuroleptics		
Divalproex sodium	Depakote	250 mg BID, up to 1250 mg/day
Miscellaneous		
Cyproheptadine	Periactin	4-16 mg daily
Ergotamine tartrate with phenobarbital and Bellafoline	Bellergal-S	One tablet BID
Methysergide maleate	Sansert	2 mg TID
Menstrual Migraine Therapy		
Fenoprofen calcium	Nalfon	600 mg TID*
Naproxen sodium	Anaprox, Naprelan	250 mg TID*
Ketoprofen	Orudis	75 mg TID*
* These drugs should be started 2 days prior to and continued through menses.		

- NSAIDs
- Alpha agonists
- Antidepressants
- Cyproheptadine.

β-*Blockers*

The β-blockers have been used successfully in the treatment of migraine headaches. It is suggested that those β-blockers that do not possess intrinsic sympathomimetic activity (ISA) are more effective than those β-blocking agents that do possess ISA. Two of these agents have received approval for the indication of migraine prophylaxis:
- Propranolol (Inderal)
- Timolol (Blocadren).

Propranolol is the agent of choice in migraine prophylaxis. It is especially useful in migraine patients with concomitant:

- Hypertension
- Angina pectoris
- Thyrotoxicosis.

Propranolol is contraindicated in patients with:

- Asthma
- Chronic obstructive lung disease
- Congestive heart failure
- Atrioventricular conduction disturbances.

This drug should be avoided in patients on concomitant therapy with:

- Insulin
- Oral hypoglycemics
- MAOIs.

The usual dose is 20 mg to 40 mg, 4 times per day. A long-acting form of propranolol (Inderal LA) is now available for once-a-day administration. This preparation enhances patient compliance.

Similar to propranolol, timolol is a nonselective β-blocker that does not possess ISA. The usual dose is 5 mg to 30 mg daily.

Other β-blockers have demonstrated efficacy in migraine prophylaxis but have not received approval for the migraine indication:

- Nadolol (Corgard)
- Atenolol (Tenormin)
- Metoprolol (Lopressor).

In selecting the appropriate β-blocker for migraine prophylaxis, it should be noted that the nonselective β-blockers have been used more successfully in migraine therapy than the cardioselective β-blockers. Also, if the patient has been refractory to two or more β-blockers, treatment with another β-blocker should not be attempted.

Nadolol is a nonselective β-blocker that is devoid of ISA and that has demonstrated efficacy in migraine.

Atenolol and metoprolol are cardioselective β-blockers which have been used effectively in migraine. These drugs may be used for migraine patients with concomitant asthma.

Methysergide

Methysergide (Sansert) is a lysergic acid derivative which is closely related to the ergot alkaloids. Its effectiveness is believed linked to blocking the inflammatory and vasoconstrictor effects of 5-HT. Long-term therapy with methysergide is associated with severe side effects. Therefore, methysergide should only be used in select patients who have been refractory to other forms of therapy.

With long-term therapy, there is a risk of fibrotic syndromes, including cardiac, pulmonary and retroperitoneal. Patients receiving methysergide should be evaluated monthly to rule out these fibrotic complications. After 6 months of continuous treatment with methysergide, an intravenous pyelogram should be performed. Methysergide should be limited to 6 months continuous treatment, followed by a 4- to 6-week drug hiatus between periods of therapy. The following side effects have been reported:

- Gastrointestinal symptoms
- Central nervous system symptoms
- Dermatological manifestations
- Edema
- Weight gain
- Hematological manifestations
- Weakness
- Arthralgia
- Myalgia.

The usual dose of methysergide is 4 mg to 8 mg per day. It is contraindicated in patients with:

- Peptic ulcer
- Pregnancy
- Thrombophlebitis
- Peripheral or coronary vascular disease
- Severe arteriosclerosis
- Severe hypertension
- Cellulitis of the lower limbs
- Pulmonary disease
- Collagen disease or fibrotic processes
- Impaired liver or renal function
- Valvular heart disease
- Debilitated states and serious infections.

Calcium Channel Blockers

If one believes that the pathogenesis of migraine is vascular in etiology, then the use of the calcium channel blockers with their suggested role in intracranial vasoconstriction may be appropriate. The calcium channel blockers that have been used effectively in migraine include:

- Nimodipine (Nimotop)
- Verapamil (Calan, Isoptin, Verelan).

These agents have not received approval for the indication of migraine treatment. Research continues into their use in migraine therapy.

Nimodipine has the highest marked selectivity for cerebral vasculature. The relative high cost of this drug has thwarted its popular prescribing.

Verapamil also has antiplatelet effects that add to its efficacy in migraine. This calcium channel blocker is noted for its long-term effects in decreasing the frequency, severity and durations of migraine. The most commonly reported side effect associated with verapamil is constipation.

Two other calcium channel blockers have been investigated for use in migraine prophylaxis, but the results were not clinically significant:

- Diltiazem (Cardizem)
- Nifedipine (Procardia).

Neuroleptics

Divalproex sodium (Depakote) is the latest agent to be approved for the indication of migraine prophylaxis. Side effects include:

- Drowsiness
- Sedation
- Ataxia
- Anorexia
- Nausea
- Vomiting.

Central nervous system side effects occur infrequently, and will usually respond to a decrease in dosage. In approximately 10% of patients, a dose-related hand tremor may present but is usually not severe enough to terminate treatment. Hair loss and alterations in liver enzymes may occur.

Nonsteroidal Anti-inflammatory Agents

The NSAIDs have been successfully used in migraine prophylaxis due to their effects on the prostaglandins and inhibition of inflammation. Several NSAIDs have been effective agents in migraine prophylaxis:

- Naproxen (Naprosyn, Naprelan)
- Aspirin
- Ketoprofen (Orudis)
- Tolmetin sodium (Tolectin)
- Fenoprofen calcium (Nalfon).

Alpha Agonist

Clonidine (Catapres-TTS) is an antihypertensive agent which has also been used in migraine prophylaxis. It has not received approval for this indication. Some studies have noted its efficacy in treating patients whose migraine attacks are triggered by tyramine-containing foods. This drug acts centrally by inhibiting sympathetic outflow from the vasomotor center in the medulla and acts peripherally by reducing the response of blood vessels to both vasoconstrictor and vasodilator substances.

The usual dose of clonidine is 0.1 mg twice daily, which may increase slowly to a daily maximum of 2.4 mg per day. Side effects of clonidine therapy are mild and include:

- Drowsiness
- Dry mouth
- Constipation
- Occasional disturbance of ejaculation.

As with propranolol, it should not be stopped abruptly due to the risk of severe hypertensive crises.

Antidepressants

The antidepressants have been investigated for the past 3 decades for use in migraine prophylaxis. The efficacy of these drugs is believed to be independent of their antidepressant actions and may be due to possible analgesic effects. Antidepressants that have been used in migraine prophylaxis include:

- Tricyclic antidepressants
- MAOIs.

These drugs are discussed in Chapter 6, *Tension-type Headaches/Coexisting Migraine and Tension-type Headaches*.

Cyproheptadine

Cyproheptadine (Periactin) is an antihistamine with mild to moderate antiserotonin activity. Cyproheptadine has been used successfully in childhood migraine although it has not demonstrated significant effects in adults with migraine. The usual dose for children is 4 mg at bedtime, and in adults, the dose is 4 mg 4 times per day up to 32 mg per day. This drug has not received approval for this indication.

■ Status Migraine

A migraine that continues over 24 hours is attributed to a sterile inflammation surrounding the enlarged vessel. Two forms of therapy for prolonged or status migraine have been noted as effective:
- Corticosteroids
- DHE.

The corticosteroids are used because of their effect on inflammation. Dexamethasone long-acting (Decadron LA) in doses of 16 mg IM will sometimes resolve the prolonged attack.

Recently, the use of DHE, administered IV with metoclopramide (Reglan), has been gaining acceptance for the treatment of status migraine. This combination therapy is administered every 8 hours for 2 days, not to exceed 2 mL per day, with excellent results. Research continues into the use of this therapy for status migraine.

■ Menstrual Migraine

For the treatment of menstrual migraine, the NSAIDs are indicated. This therapy is started 2 days before menses and continued through the menstrual flow. The NSAIDs used in menstrual migraine include:
- Fenoprofen calcium (Nalfon)
- Naproxen sodium (Anaprox)
- Mefenamic acid (Ponstel).

Biofeedback

The use of biofeedback in migraine treatment has offered an excellent adjunct to pharmacological therapy and can be used in those patients unable to use medications. Biofeedback training traces its origins to the discipline of self-awareness. By using a monitoring device, the patient is taught to control autonomic functions that previously were considered strictly involuntary actions including:

- Blood flow
- Blood pressure
- Pulse.

The training is achieved through the reinforcement of the correct response to a conditioned stimulus. Biofeedback training utilizes:

- Relaxation methods
- Imagery
- Use of self-hypnotic phrases.

The use of biofeedback training in headache therapy is focused on two types of biofeedback:

- Temperature training
- Muscle relaxation (EMG) training.

Temperature training focuses on the patient increasing the local peripheral temperature of the hand and, thereby, redirecting blood flow to that area. Autogenic phrases (Table 4.4) which focus on warmth and relaxation are practiced while the patient's finger temperature is being monitored. Patients may also focus on warm images, such as sitting by a fire or on a beach, holding a hot cup of tea, etc. By utilizing these techniques at the first sign of a headache, it is hoped that the patient can abort the acute attack or, at least, decrease the severity and duration of the migraine headache.

TABLE 4.4 — TEMPERATURE TRAINING PHRASES

I feel quite quiet...

I am beginning to feel quite relaxed...

My feet feel heavy and relaxed...

My ankles, my knees and my hips feel heavy, relaxed and comfortable...

My solar plexus, and the whole central portion of my body feel relaxed and quiet...

My hands, my arms and my shoulders feel heavy, relaxed and comfortable...

My neck, my jaw and my forehead feel relaxed — they feel comfortable and smooth...

My whole body feels quiet, heavy, comfortable and relaxed.

I am quite relaxed...

My arms and hands are heavy and warm...

I feel quite quiet...

My whole body is relaxed and my hands are warm — relaxed and warm.

My hands are warm...
Warmth is flowing into my hands, they are warm... warm.

Muscle relaxation training involves the use of an EMG monitor that measures muscle tension over a particular area, such as the:

- Forehead
- Neck
- Shoulder.

Tension is measured via a high pitched tone which increases as the muscles tense and decreases as the tension is reduced. To achieve this decrease in tension, a set of progressive relaxation exercises are employed (Table 4.5). Patients are encouraged to practice these exercises at least twice daily to help them identify which muscles are being tensed at times of stress or during a headache. The use of EMG biofeedback at the time of an acute migraine will hopefully decrease the severity of the headache and possibly prevent attacks from occurring.

REFERENCES

Diamond S, Freitag FG, Diamond ML, Urban GJ, Pepper B, Bhambhvani D. Open-label long-term use of divalproex sodium in headache. *Headache Q*. 1997;8:42-44.

Dihydroergotamine Nasal Spray Multicenter Investigators. Efficacy, safety, and tolerability of dihydroergotamine nasal spray as monotherapy in the treatment of acute migraine. *Headache*. 1995;35:177-184.

Ferrari MD, Haan J. Acute treatment of migraine attacks. *Curr Opin Neurol*. 1995;8:237-242.

Fozard JR. 5-HT in migraine: evidence from 5-HT receptor antagonists for a neuronal etiology. In: Sandler M, Collins GM (eds). *Migraine: A Spectrum of Ideas*. Oxford, England: Oxford University Press; 1990:128-141.

Fozard JR. The pharmacological basis of migraine treatment. In: Blau JN (ed). *Migraine. Clinical and Research Aspects*. Baltimore, Md: Johns Hopkins University Press; 1987:165-184.

Gallagher RM. Acute treatment of migraine with dihydroergotamine nasal spray. Dihydroergotamine Working Group. *Arch Neurol*. 1996;53:1285-1291.

Hering R, Kuritzky A. Sodium valproate in the prophylactic treatment of migraine: a double-blind study versus placebo. *Cephalalgia*. 1992;12:81-84.

Klapper JA, Stanton J. Clinical experience with patient administered subcutaneous dihydroergotamine mesylate in refractory headaches. *Headache*. 1992;32:21-23.

Kumar KL. Recent advances in the acute management of migraine and cluster headaches. *J Gen Intern Med*. 1994;9:339-348.

Maizels M, Scott B, Cohen W, Chen W. Intranasal lidocaine for treatment of migraine: a randomized, double-blind, controlled trial. *JAMA*. 1996;276:319-321.

Moskowitz MA. Neurogenic versus vascular mechanisms of sumatriptan and ergot alkaloids in migraine. *Trends Pharmacol Sci*. 1992;13:307-311.

Peroutka SJ. Developments in 5-hydroxytryptamine receptor pharmacology in migraine. *Neurol Clin*. 1990;8:829-838.

Plosker GL, McTavish D. Sumatriptan. A reappraisal of its pharmacology and therapeutic efficacy in the acute treatment of migraine and cluster headache. *Drugs*. 1994;47:622-651.

Raskin NH. Headache. *West J Med*. 1994;161(special issue):299-302.

Raskin NH. Repetitive intravenous dihydroergotamine as therapy for intractable migraine. *Neurology*. 1986;36:995-997.

Saadah HA. Abortive headache therapy with intramuscular dihydroergotamine. *Headache*. 1992;32:18-20.

Salonen R, Ashford E, Dahlïof C, et al. Intranasal sumatriptan for the acute treatment of migraine. International Intranasal Sumatriptan Study Group. *J Neurol*. 1994;241:463-469.

Tfelt-Hansen P. Drug treatment of migraine: acute treatment and migraine prophylaxis. *Curr Opin Neurol*. 1996;9:211-213.

Ziegler D, Ford R, Kriegler J, et al. Dihydroergotamine nasal spray for the acute treatment of migraine. *Neurology*. 1994;44:447-453.

4

TABLE 4.5 — EMG FEEDBACK EXERCISES

Relaxation of Facial Area With Neck, Shoulders and Upper Back

Let all your muscles go loose and heavy. Just settle back quietly and comfortably.

Wrinkle up your forehead now; wrinkle and smooth it out. Picture the entire forehead and scalp becoming smoother as the relaxation increases...

Now frown and crease your brows and study the tension...

Let go of the tension again.

Smooth out the forehead once more...

Now, close your eyes tighter and tighter.

Feel the tension... and relax your eyes.

Keep your eyes closed, gently, comfortably, and notice the relaxation...

Now clench your jaw, bite your teeth together; study the tension throughout the jaw...

Relax your jaw now. Let your lips part slightly...

Appreciate the relaxation...

Now press your tongue hard against the roof of your mouth. Look for the tension.

All right, let your tongue return to a comfortable and relaxed position...

Now purse your lips, press your lips together tighter and tighter.

Relax the lips. Note the contrast between tension and relaxation. Feel the relaxation all over your face, all over your forehead and scalp, eyes, jaws, lips, tongue and neck muscles.

Press your head back as far as it can go and feel the tension in the neck; roll it to the right and feel the tension shift; now roll it to the left.

Straighten your head and bring it forward and press your chin against your chest.

Let your head return to a comfortable position and study the relaxation. Let the relaxation develop…

Shrug your shoulders up. Hold the tension…

Drop your shoulders and feel the relaxation. Neck and shoulders relaxed…

Shrug your shoulders again and move them around. Bring your shoulders up and forward and back. Feel the tension in your shoulders up and forward and back.

Drop your shoulders once more and relax. Let the relaxation spread deep into the shoulders, right into your back muscles; relax your neck and throat, and your jaws and other facial areas as the pure relaxation takes over and grows deeper… deeper… ever deeper…

4

5

Cluster Headaches

Cluster headaches have been known by many names, including:

- Horton's headache
- Ciliary or migrainous neuralgia
- Histaminic cephalalgia
- Vidian and Sluder's neuralgia.

In 1952, Charles Kunkle and his colleagues coined the term "cluster headache" which is characteristic of the periodicity of these headaches which will present in a series or the so-called cluster periods.

The Classification Committee of the International Headache Society (IHS) has defined cluster headaches as:

Attacks of severe, strictly unilateral pain, orbitally, supraorbitally and/or temporally, lasting 15 to 180 minutes and occurring from once every other day to 8 times a day.

The criteria established for episodic cluster headaches note that these headaches occur in periods lasting 7 days to 1 year, divided by pain-free periods lasting 14 days or more. Chronic cluster headaches are characterized by the frequency of the attacks which occur for more than 1 year without remission or with remissions lasting less than 14 days.

The associated symptoms of cluster headaches include:

- Conjunctival injection
- Lacrimation
- Nasal congestion
- Rhinorrhea
- Sweating and facial flushing on the ipsilateral side
- Partial Horner's syndrome.

The pain of cluster headaches is noted for its intense severity. It is described as:
- Throbbing or pulsating
- Severe
- Constant.

Some patients will depict the pain as sharp, knife-like or stabbing sensations into the eye. The excruciating nature of the pain has prompted patients to attempt or actually commit suicide. Patients will desire to be upright and moving during an acute attack, as opposed to a migraine patient who prefers to be quiet and resting during a severe attack.

Duration of acute cluster headache attacks is noted for its brevity, lasting from a few minutes up to 4 hours. Patients will experience one to several attacks per day during a series. Many patients will be awakened at the same time each night.

The cluster periods occur most frequently in the spring and fall. During a cluster series, the patient will note that alcohol will trigger an acute attack, although it will have no effect during a remission period.

Cluster headaches, as opposed to migraine, are primarily a male disorder. Prevalence rate in males is believed to be ten to one. The onset of cluster usually occurs between the ages of 20 to 40 years. There is an infrequent reporting of a hereditary history of cluster headaches. Table 5.1 compares the features of cluster and migraine headaches.

Abortive Therapy

Figure 5.1 offers the options available in the treatment of cluster headaches. The characteristic limited duration of acute cluster headaches limits the number of agents used in abortive therapy. These agents include:

- Oxygen
- Ergotamine tartrate
- Dihydroergotamine
- Sumatriptan
- Intranasal lidocaine
- Intranasal cocaine.

Oxygen inhalation at 7 L/minute, by facial mask for 10 to 15 minutes, has demonstrated efficacy in abortive therapy of acute cluster headaches. The ergotamine tartrate preparations may be effective in some patients and, in combination with caffeine, is available in oral and rectal preparations. Due to the brief duration of the acute attack, the rapid absorption of ergotamine tartrate in the sublingual preparation may be indicated for the cluster headache patient. Contraindications for ergotamine preparations have been reviewed in Chapter 4, *Migraine Headaches*.

The rapid absorption of parenteral dihydroergotamine may provide rapid relief of the acute cluster attacks. The promising results of intranasal dihydroergotamine in migraine abortive therapy extends to its use in acute cluster headaches.

Sumatriptan has also shown efficacy for cluster abortive therapy. The rapid onset of action with subcutaneous sumatriptan enhances its benefits in acute cluster headaches. The short half-life (2 hours) of oral sumatriptan precludes its use in acute cluster headache. Intranasal sumatriptan, with an initially higher plasma concentration than its oral preparation, would indicate it to be more effective in the management of acute cluster headaches.

Investigators have documented good response from the intranasal application of lidocaine or cocaine. Kittrelle's group examined the use of a 4% lidocaine solution applied by nasal dropper into the nostril ipsilateral to the headache. For patients with nasal congestion that complicated the procedure, 0.5% phenyle-

TABLE 5.1 — CONTRASTING FEATURES OF MIGRAINE AND CLUSTER HEADACHES		
Feature	Migraine	Cluster
Pain site	Unilateral, occasionally bilateral	Always unilateral, periorbital
Frequency of attacks	1 to 8/month	1 to 6/day, during a series
Duration of attacks	4 to 48 hours	10 minutes to 3 hours
Occurrence of attacks	Intermittent, 2 to 8/month	Daily for several weeks to months
Seasonal occurrence	No relationship	Occurs more frequently in spring and fall
Age at onset	10 to 40 years	20 to 50 years
Sex incidence	65% to 70% female	90% male
Family history of headaches	90%	7%
Prodromes	25% to 30% of cases	Absent
Nausea and vomiting	85%	2% to 5%
Blurred vision	Frequent	Infrequent

Ptosis	1% to 2%		30%
Lacrimation	Infrequent		Frequent
Polyuria	90%		2%
Nasal congestion	Uncommon		70%
Miosis	Absent		50%
Chemical Changes			
Decrease in plasma serotonin	80%		None
Rise in plasma histamine	None		90%
Rise in CSF acetylcholine	None		30%
Abbreviations: CSF, cerebrospinal fluid.			

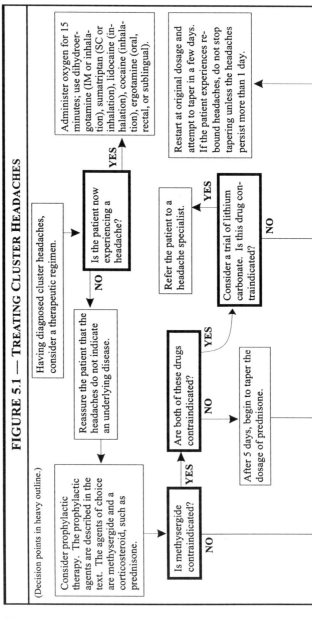

FIGURE 5.1 — TREATING CLUSTER HEADACHES

(Decision points in heavy outline.)

Having diagnosed cluster headaches, consider a therapeutic regimen.

Is the patient now experiencing a headache?

YES → Administer oxygen for 15 minutes; use dihydroergotamine (IM or inhalation), sumatriptan (SC or inhalation), lidocaine (inhalation), cocaine (inhalation), ergotamine (oral, rectal, or sublingual).

NO → Reassure the patient that the headaches do not indicate an underlying disease.

Consider prophylactic therapy. The prophylactic agents are described in the text. The agents of choice are methysergide and a corticosteroid, such as prednisone.

Is methysergide contraindicated?

NO

YES → Are both of these drugs contraindicated?

NO → After 5 days, begin to taper the dosage of prednisone.

YES → Consider a trial of lithium carbonate. Is this drug contraindicated?

YES → Refer the patient to a headache specialist.

NO

Restart at original dosage and attempt to taper in a few days. If the patient experiences rebound headaches, do not stop tapering unless the headaches persist more than 1 day.

96

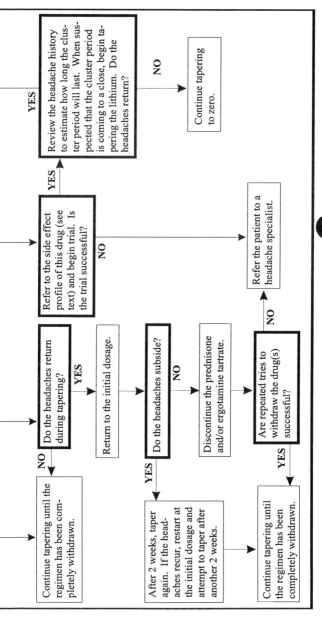

phrine hydrochloride was used prior to the lidocaine application. Robbins has confirmed this early report by describing the successful use of 4 sprays of the 4% solution. Barré and colleagues investigated the use of intranasal cocaine hydrochloride in a saline solution. The solution was applied to the sphenopalatine fossa region from 15 seconds to 3 minutes. Dependency problems were not reported in either study.

Pain relief measures may also be considered. However, the acute attack may have subsided by the time the patient reaches a physician's office or emergency department to receive an analgesic. The use of transnasal butorphanol may offer a rapid, easily administered alternative to parenteral analgesics.

Topical capsaicin has been available over the counter for pain relief for several years. However, intranasal capsaicin is a recent newcomer to cluster headache treatment. Although capsaicin does not affect the headache process, it may relieve the acute pain. Intranasal capsaicin appears to be more effective in patients with episodic cluster than chronic cluster headache. In the author's clinical experience, the results of this therapy have not been promising.

Prophylactic Therapy

Table 5.2 reviews both abortive and prophylactic agents used in cluster therapy. The goal of prophylactic therapy is to limit the length of the cluster period and decrease the severity of the attacks that occur. Agents of choice in the prophylactic therapy of episodic cluster headaches are:

- Methysergide
- Corticosteroids.

Methysergide is used for prophylactic therapy for severe and/or frequent, uncontrollable vascular headaches and is believed to be effective in vascular head-aches due to its selective vasoconstrictive effects as well as its mild anti-inflammatory effects. The usual dose is 2 mg 3 times per day. Because of its potential for serious side effects, methysergide is not indicated for long-term therapy. Continuous use of methy-sergide has been linked to retroperitoneal, cardiac and pulmonary fibrosis. Gastrointestinal symptoms, CNS, dermatological manifestations, edema, weight gain, hematological manifestations, weakness, arthralgia and myalgia have also been reported.

During therapy with this agent, the patient should be examined frequently for evidence of fibrotic con-ditions. Patients treated with methysergide for 6 months must undergo a 6 to 8 week drug hiatus. At the end of a 6-month interval of methysergide treat-ment, the patient should undergo an intravenous pyelo-gram (IVP). Because of the self-limiting nature of episodic cluster headaches, methysergide can be con-sidered for prophylactic therapy.

The anti-inflammatory effects of the corticoster-oids probably explain their effective use in cluster pro-phylaxis. Although long-term therapy with these agents is not encouraged due to the potential for ser-ious, prolonged side effects, the corticosteroids are used for short-term cluster therapy. Prednisone and methylprednisolone are often used for cluster treat-ment. These drugs are gradually tapered over 6 to 8 weeks and then discontinued.

Chronic cluster headaches represent a complex therapeutic problem for the treating physician. Agents used in the treatment of chronic cluster headaches in-clude:
- Lithium carbonate
- Calcium channel blockers
- Histamine desensitization.

TABLE 5.2 — THERAPY OF CLUSTER HEADACHES

	Generic (Trade) Name	Route	Dosage
PROPHYLACTIC TREATMENT	Methysergide maleate (Sansert)	Oral	2 mg TID.
	Prednisone	Oral	40 mg/day in divided doses (to be tapered slowly).
	Methylprednisolone (Medrol)	Oral	16 mg every other day.
	Ergotamine tartrate with phenobarbital and Bellafoline (Bellergal-S)	Oral	One tablet BID.
	Lithium carbonate (Eskalith, Lithane, Lithobid)	Oral	300 mg TID (serum levels should be closely monitored to prevent toxicity).
	Verapamil (Calan, Isoptin, Verelan)	Oral	240 mg per day.

Oxygen 100%	Inhalation	By face mask, at 7 L/minute for 15 minutes PRN.
Dihydroergotamine (D.H.E. 45)	Intramuscular	1 mg at hourly intervals, up to 3 mg/ day.
Dihydroergotamine	Intranasal	2 mg, one spray in each nostril; may repeat in 15 minutes, up to four treatments per day.
Sumatriptan (Imitrex)	Subcutaneous	6 mg at onset; may repeat dose in 1 hour, up to 12 mg/day.
Sumatriptan	Intranasal	20 mg, one spray in one nostril at onset; may repeat within 2 to 24 hours, limited to two sprays per day.
Lidocaine 4% (Xylocaine)	Intranasal	1 mL (15 to 16 drops) to affected nostril, repeat in 5 minutes PRN, maximum 4 times per day; if nasal congestion is present, use 0.5% phenylephrine (Neo-Synephrine) nasal solution 3 to 5 minutes before instilling lidocaine.
Cocaine HCl 10%	Intranasal	Two drops into affected nostril or both nostrils, 4 times/day PRN.
Ergotamine tartrate with caffeine (Cafergot, Wigraine)	Oral	Two tablets immediately at onset; may repeat every 1/2 hour, up to six per day.
(Cafergot)	Rectal	Insert one suppository immediately at onset; may repeat in 1 hour, if necessary up to two suppositories per day.
Ergotamine (Ergostat)	Sublingual	One tablet at onset; may repeat every 30 minutes, up to three tablets per day, five tablets per week.

ABORTIVE TREATMENT

■ Lithium Carbonate

Lithium carbonate has been demonstrated by both Ekbom and Kudrow as effective therapy in chronic cluster headaches. Although the method of action of lithium in this disorder is not fully understood, some investigators have attributed this efficacy to alteration of electrical conductivity in the central nervous system. The usual dosage of lithium is 300 mg 3 times per day. To avoid toxicity, the serum lithium level should be monitored every 4 to 6 weeks and maintained between 0.5 to 1.5 Meq/L. If the patient's drug levels cannot be easily monitored, another therapeutic agent should be considered. Transient, mild side effects associated with lithium therapy include:

- Thirst
- Polyuria
- Fatigue
- Tremor.

■ Calcium Channel Blockers

The calcium channel blockers have been recognized as effective in the treatment of both episodic and chronic cluster headaches. The action of these agents in cluster headaches is not attributed to an effect on vascular dilation. Researchers have implicated the blockade of the release of the pain-inducing neurotransmitters, such as substance P which has been identified in the pathogenesis of cluster headaches. Substance P is dependent on calcium for its release. Verapamil and nimodipine have been investigated in cluster prophylaxis.

■ Histamine Desensitization

Histamine desensitization has been used in the treatment of patients with chronic cluster headaches who are refractory to other forms of therapy. The therapy is administered via an intravenous solution combined with histamine phosphate. This treatment is best undertaken in an inpatient setting, the patient to be closely monitored for effects from the therapy. Treatment can be concluded in 9 to 11 days.

Although histamine desensitization has not gained in popularity for the treatment of cluster headache, it is a viable and safe alternative. During therapy, if the patient experiences headache, facial flushing, or throbbing, "sensitization," instead of desensitization, may be occurring. In such cases, the next dosage should be reduced by one-half, and subsequently build it up again to immediately below the level at which the reaction started.

In a recent study at the Inpatient Diamond Headache Clinic in Chicago, improvement was noted in 48 of 59 patients. The treatment protocol for IV Histamine Desensitization at the inpatient unit of the Diamond Headache Clinic is as follows:

- Day 1: 2.75 mg of histamine phosphate is used in a slow drip lasting 8 hours
- Days 2 through 11: the patient receives two bottles each day containing histamine phosphate 5.5 mg in each bottle (total of 21 bottles)
  - Start each bottle at the rate of 20 cc/hour
  - Increase by 10 cc/hour every 15 to 30 minutes until patient experiences symptoms of flushing or stuffiness (not to exceed 125 cc/hour)
  - Titrate the drip rate according to the patient's tolerance. If the patient develops symptoms of headache, decrease the IV rate immediately.

■ **Surgical Intervention**

For patients refractory to all types of therapy, surgical intervention may be considered. Some surgical procedures have been abandoned such as:

- Resection of the greater superficial petrosal nerve

- Section of the nervous intermedius
- Ablation of the sphenopalatine ganglion.

Recently, procedures involving the trigeminal ganglion have been proposed. These procedures include:
- Partial trigeminal root section (posterior approach)
- Percutaneous radiofrequency gangliorhizolysis
- Glycerol injections of the trigeminal cistern
- Posterior fossa trigeminal sensory rhizotomy.

Surgical therapy for chronic cluster headaches should only be considered for those patients who have not responded to any conventional form of therapy.

Other Forms of Cluster Headaches

Investigators have described other forms of cluster headaches that may occur. Cluster headaches and chronic paroxysmal hemicrania (CPH) have been identified by the Classification Committee of the IHS as sharing the following characteristics:
- Unilaterality of the pain
- Severe intensity of the pain
- Location of the pain
- Accompanying autonomic phenomena
- Temporal pattern of the attacks.

Features that distinguish these two disorders are:
- Sex preponderance (female dominance in CPH)
- Frequency and duration of attacks
- Night preponderance
- Drug effects (symptomatic and prophylactic).

Chronic paroxysmal hemicrania is noted for the excessive daily frequency of the attacks, 15 or more per day. The brief duration of the attacks (described as jabs) is also diagnostic. The severity of the attacks is intense, and the pain can be triggered by certain movements, such as bending the head forward. Sjaastad has noted that the response of these patients to treatment with indomethacin is a highly distinctive feature. The dosage ranges from 12.5 to 250 mg per day. CPH is a rarely occurring disorder, with approximately 80 documented cases throughout the world.

In contrast, cluster headache variant is very prevalent. Three types of pain are associated with cluster headache variant, although the disorder may present in different combinations in individual patients. These combinations include:

- *Atypical cluster headache*: atypical location, duration and frequency occurring several times per day.
- *Multiple jabs*: sharp, variable pains that last only a few seconds and occur several times per day. (These pains can be triggered by certain head movements.)
- *Background vascular headache*: chronic, continuous usually sharply localized (often unilateral). These headaches vary in severity and may be throbbing or become throbbing during exertion.

These patients also demonstrated a notable response to indomethacin therapy. Patients refractory to indomethacin have been successfully treated with antidepressants or lithium due to a secondary depression. Sjaastad's group has described cluster variant headache as "hemicrania continua."

REFERENCES

Barré F. Cocaine as an abortive agent in cluster headache. *Headache*. 1982;22:69-73.

Diamond S. Head pain. Diagnosis and management. *Clin Symp.* 1994;46:2-34.

Diamond S, Freitag FG, Bhambhvani S. IV histamine desensitization therapy in recidivist chronic cluster headache patients. *Cephalalgia.* 1997;17:456. Abstract.

Ekbom K. Treatment of cluster headache: clinical trials, design and results. *Cephalalgia.* 1995;15(suppl 15):33-36.

Fusco BM, Marabini S, Maggi CA, Fiore G, Geppetti P. Preventative effect of repeated nasal applications of capsaicin in cluster headache. *Pain.* 1994;59:321-325.

Headache Classification Committee of the International Headache Society. Classification and diagnostic criteria for headache disorders, cranial neuralgias and facial pain. *Cephalalgia.* 1988;8(suppl 7):1-96.

Kittrelle JP, Grouse DS, Seybold ME. Cluster headache. Local anesthetic abortive agents. *Arch Neurol.* 1985;42:496-498.

Kudrow L. Cluster headache: diagnosis, management, and treatment. In: Dalessio DJ, Silberstein SD (eds). *Wolff's Headache and Other Head Pain.* 6th ed. New York, NY: Oxford University Press; 1993:171-197.

Kunkle EC, Pfeiffer JB Jr, Wilhoit WM, Hamrich LW Jr. Recurrent brief headaches in "cluster" pattern. *Trans Am Neurol Assoc.* 1952;77:240-241.

Medina JL, Diamond S. Cluster headache variant. Spectrum of a new syndrome. *Arch Neurol.* 1981;38:705-709.

Rapoport AM, Sheftell FD. Intranasal medications for the treatment of migraine and cluster headache. *CNS Drugs.* 1997;7:37-45.

Robbins L. Intranasal lidocaine for cluster headache. *Headache.* 1995;35:83-84.

Sjaastad O. Chronic paroxysmal hemicrania: clinical aspects and controversies. In: *Migraine: Clinical, Therapeutic, Conceptual and Research Aspects.* London: Chapman and Hall; 1987:135-152.

Wilkinson M, Pfaffenrath V, Schoenen J. Diener HC, Steiner TJ. Migraine and cluster headache—their management with sumatriptan: a critical review of the current clinical experience. *Cephalalgia.* 1995;15:337-357.

6

Tension-type Headaches/ Coexisting Migraine and Tension-type Headaches

Tension-type Headaches

The terms "muscle contraction" or "tension" headaches have been used interchangeably for several years. The Classification Committee of the International Headache Society (IHS) has established the term "tension-type" headache as the correct label for these headaches.

The tension-type headache is a manifestation of the body's reaction to:
- Stress
- Anxiety
- Depression
- Emotional conflicts
- Fatigue
- Repressed hostility.

The physiological response includes:
- Reflex dilatation of the external cranial vessels
- Contraction of the skeletal muscles of the:
  - Head
  - Neck
  - Face.

Tension-type headaches are defined by the Classification Committee of the IHS as recurrent episodes of headache lasting minutes to days. Pain is usually:
- A pressure or tightening sensation
- Of mild to moderate severity
- Bilateral in location

- Not exacerbated by physical activity
- Associated symptoms are not prominent.

Tension-type headaches are identified as being either episodic or chronic. The distinguishing feature between the two types is the frequency of chronic tension-type headaches to be at least 15 days per month for at least 6 months.

These headaches are dominant in females and can occur at any age. Typically, the headaches start between the ages of 20 to 40 years. A family history of similar headaches may be noted. The pain is described as steady and nonpulsating and may be depicted as:
- Bitemporal or bioccipital tightness
- Band-like sensations around the head
- Viselike ache
- A weight
- Pressure sensations
- Drawing
- Soreness.

The site of the headache is primarily the:
- Forehead
- Temples
- Back of the head or neck.

Other locations may be affected and are usually bilateral, as opposed to migraine which is usually unilateral. On palpation, nodules may be noted which are sharply localized. The pain may radiate to other areas, such as the neck or shoulders. Shivering or exposure to the cold may exacerbate the pain.

Patients with episodic, tension-type headaches rarely consult a physician for their attacks and often treat themselves successfully with over-the-counter (OTC) analgesics. When these are not effective, combination analgesics such as aspirin plus butalbital and caffeine (Fiorinal); acetaminophen with butalbital

(Phrenilin); or acetaminophen plus butalbital and caffeine (Fioricet, Esgic) may be prescribed. If more pain-relieving potency is required, a compound agent with aspirin or acetaminophen plus butalbital, caffeine and codeine may be considered (Fiorinal/Fioricet with Codeine). Esgic, Fioricet and Fioricet with Codeine are aspirin-free and avoid any aspirin-related GI problems. When used properly, these products are highly effective with little chance of abuse or habituation.

Chronic tension-type headaches are continuous or unremitting. These patients will present with prolonged histories of headaches. These headaches are often a manifestation of an underlying psychologic conflict, such as anxiety or depression. The examining physician should review any family, work, school or marital conflicts. If the patient is not forthcoming with this information, the review may need to take place over several visits. The psychological inventory should include questions about the following:

- Life stresses
- Occupation
- Habits
- Personality traits
- Marital relations
- Social relationships
- Sexual problems
- Methods of coping with stress.

The patient with chronic anxiety usually:

- Reports only one type of headache
- Describes headache as annoying and not associated with other symptoms, such as nausea and vomiting
- Complains of difficulty falling asleep, which is the feature that distinguishes anxiety from depression.

Because these patients will worry excessively about their headaches, reassurance is a prominent aspect of their therapy.

In patients with chronic tension-type headaches associated with depression, a variety of symptoms may be present in addition to the headaches. Physical symptoms include:

- Sleep disturbance—early or frequent awakening
- Shortness of breath
- Constipation
- Weight loss
- Fatigue
- Decreased sexual drive
- Palpations
- Menstrual changes.

The patient with underlying depression may look "blue" and in low spirits during the interview. Spontaneous crying may occur. Emotional complaints include:

- Feelings of guilt
- Hopelessness
- Unworthiness
- Basic fear of insanity
- Rumination over the past, present and future
- Fear of physical disease or death.

Patients may note that morning is the worst time of day and, similar to depression, a diurnal variation may be identified with their pain. Psychic complaints are:

- Poor concentration
- Loss of interest
- Low or no ambition
- Indecisiveness
- Poor memory
- Suicidal ideation.

The patient may relate the onset of the headaches to a specific event, such as an accident. The patient will relate the headaches to a bodily injury or alteration, although physical and radiological examination will rule out these conditions. The patient may relate the headaches to the death of a loved one, a minor illness, an injection, surgical procedure, loss of a job, or a divorce. The event may be perceived as much more serious and out of proportion to the actual occurrence or its impact.

■ Treatment

When confronted with an acute, episodic tension-type headache, relief can usually be obtained with OTC analgesics, such as:

- Aspirin
- Acetaminophen
- Ibuprofen
- Naproxen sodium
- Ketoprofen.

Caffeine has demonstrated efficacy as an analgesic adjuvant in the treatment of tension-type headache. In a recent study, a combination agent containing ibuprofen and caffeine was used successfully in the treatment of episodic, tension-type headaches. The ibuprofen/caffeine agent is not available in the United States as yet. The amount of caffeine used in this combination is equivalent to two large cups of coffee.

For patients with chronic tension-type headache, pharmacological therapy should be prescribed cautiously. Due to the chronic nature of these headaches, addicting anxiolytic agents (such as the benzodiazepines) should be avoided. A nonaddicting anxiolytic (eg, buspirone) should be considered. Buspirone is a selective 5-HT_{1A} serotonin receptor-partial agonist with a low incidence of sedation.

Figure 6.1 provides a schematic drawing of the treatment of chronic, tension-type headaches. Due to the continuous nature of chronic, tension-type headaches, addicting analgesics should be avoided. The patient may use OTC analgesics, although caffeine-containing analgesics should also be avoided to prevent caffeine withdrawal headaches. The nonsteroidal anti-inflammatory drugs (NSAIDs) may be used successfully in the abortive therapy of these headaches.

Tricyclic antidepressants are the agents of choice in the prophylactic treatment of chronic, tension-type headaches associated with depression. These agents may be effective independent of their antidepressant actions as they have been recognized for their analgesic effects. Table 6.1 describes the various effects of the antidepressants. Selection of the antidepressant may be dependent on the presence of a sleep disturbance. Amitriptyline and doxepin are indicated for their sedative effects. Other patients who do not require a sedative effect may respond well to protriptyline. The most commonly used tricyclic antidepressants in chronic, tension-type headache therapy are:

- Amitriptyline
- Doxepin
- Protriptyline
- Nortriptyline
- Desipramine
- Imipramine.

Nontricyclic agents are the second generation of antidepressants. They are not associated with the anticholinergic effects present with the tricyclic agents. These antidepressants include:

- Maprotiline
- Trazodone
- Fluoxetine
- Bupropion.

FIGURE 6.1 — TREATING TENSION-TYPE HEADACHE

(Decision points in heavy outline.)

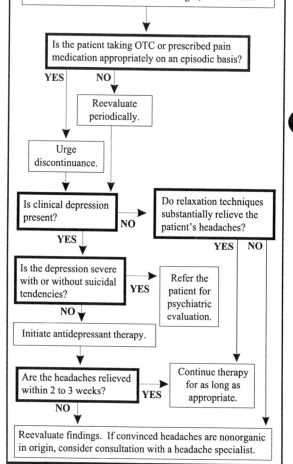

Having determined that the patient is suffering from tension-type headaches, consider ways to treat the underlying problem. Counsel the patient on coping with stress. Also consider recommending one or more of the following: relaxation exercises, neck or back massages, biofeedback.

Is the patient taking OTC or prescribed pain medication appropriately on an episodic basis?

YES | **NO**

Reevaluate periodically.

Urge discontinuance.

Is clinical depression present? → **NO** → Do relaxation techniques substantially relieve the patient's headaches?

YES

YES | **NO**

Is the depression severe with or without suicidal tendencies? **YES** → Refer the patient for psychiatric evaluation.

NO

Initiate antidepressant therapy.

Are the headaches relieved within 2 to 3 weeks? **YES** → Continue therapy for as long as appropriate.

NO

Reevaluate findings. If convinced headaches are nonorganic in origin, consider consultation with a headache specialist.

6

TABLE 6.1 — EFFECTS OF ANTIDEPRESSANTS

Drug	Serotonin Inhibition	Norepinephrine Inhibition	Dopamine Inhibition	Sedative Effects	Anticholinergic Effects
Amitriptyline	Moderate	Weak	Inactive	Strong	Strong
Bupropion	Weak	Weak	Weak	None	None
Clomipramine	Potent	Inactive	Inactive	Mild	Mild
Desipramine	Weak	Potent	Inactive	Mild	Moderate
Doxepin	Moderate	Moderate	Inactive	Strong	Strong
Fluoxetine	Potent	Weak	Inactive	None	Mild-none
Fluvoxamine	Potent	Inactive	Inactive	Mild	Mild
Imipramine	Fairly potent	Moderate	Inactive	Moderate	Strong
Maprotiline	Weak	Moderate	Inactive	Moderate	Moderate
Nefazodone	Fairly potent	Weak	Inactive	Strong	Mild
Nortriptyline	Weak	Fairly potent	Inactive	Mild	Moderate

Paroxetine	Potent	Weak	Weak	None	None
Protriptyline	Weak	Fairly potent	Inactive	None	Strong
Sertraline	Potent	Weak	Weak	None	None
Trazodone	Fairly potent	Weak	Inactive	Strong	Mild
Trimipramine	Weak	Weak	Inactive	Moderate	Moderate
Venlafaxine	Potent	Potent	Weak	Mild	Mild

6

For those patients unresponsive to the tricyclic antidepressants, the monoamine oxidase inhibitors (MAOIs) may be considered, such as phenelzine sulfate. Patients treated with MAOIs must be carefully instructed to avoid tyramine-containing foods (Table 4.1). The patient should also be advised that certain concomitant drugs should be avoided, including pressor agents and certain opiates.

Biofeedback has also demonstrated efficacy in the treatment of chronic, tension-type headaches. EMG training has been effective in decreasing the severity of acute headaches as well as diminishing the frequency of these attacks. (For further information on biofeedback and EMG training, refer to Chapter 4, *Migraine Headaches*. Table 4.5 illustrates specific dialogue used in EMG training.) Psychological counseling may be indicated for those patients with severe depression.

Coexisting Migraine and Tension-type Headaches

Some patients will experience a combination of tension-type and migraine headaches. Previously known as the mixed headache syndrome, this disorder is now identified as coexisting migraine and tension-type headaches. The following symptomatology is associated with these headaches:

- Daily, chronic, tension-type headache
- Hard or "sick" migraine-like headache
- Increased susceptibility of habituation to analgesics or ergots.

The majority of the patients with this syndrome will note a history of periodic migraine headaches, dating from adolescence or their twenties with a daily, milder form of headache occurring at a later age. Other patients will depict a history of daily headaches that occasionally presents as a harder or "sick" headache similar to migraine. They have difficulty distinguishing between the two types of headaches. Finally, a group of patients will describe a long history of migraine headaches that gradually become less vascular in nature and the frequency increases to an almost daily pattern. During the history, it is essential that the interviewer ask the patient, "How many types of headaches do you experience?"

The symptoms of each type of headache have been reviewed in their respective sections. Due to the lack of distinctive features, many patients with coexisting migraine and tension-type headaches have been misdiagnosed and treated inappropriately. They will present with long lists of treating physicians, unsuccessful treatments, and repeated admission and visits to emergency departments.

Because of the frequency of their headaches, many of these patients are habituated to analgesics, both OTC and prescribed. Many patients will be using large amounts of caffeine-containing analgesics and complain of caffeine withdrawal headaches when the drugs are stopped. Some will be consuming excessive amounts of ergotamine preparations and experience ergot rebound headaches when they attempt to discontinue the drug. Other patients may have become dependent on benzodiazepines. Before initiating treatment, it is essential that the habituating agent be discontinued.

■ Treatment

Many patients diagnosed with coexisting migraine and tension-type headaches are suffering from an underlying depression. Antidepressants have been recognized as the agents of choice for prophylactic treatment of this syndrome. Again, the antidepressants may be effective in these patients for both their antidepressant action as well as their analgesic effects.

Due to the complex nature of this syndrome, the use of combination therapy is often indicated. Although combined therapy with a tricyclic antidepressant and an MAOI was considered contraindicated, many patients with coexisting migraine and tension-type headaches have been successfully treated. Usually, these patients have been refractory to conventional forms of therapy, and the combined use of these agents is effective in treating both types of headaches. Ideally, this therapy should only be initiated in an inpatient setting at which the patient can be closely monitored for any symptoms of serious interactions between the drugs. The patient must be carefully instructed regarding the avoidance of tyramine-containing foods (Table 4.1) and drugs which interact with the MAOI. Combined therapy should only be undertaken by a physician experienced in this treatment.

Other agents may be employed in combination or co-therapy. The use of the tricyclic antidepressants in combination with propranolol or the calcium channel blockers has been effective for some patients with this syndrome. Again, initiation of this combined therapy is best undertaken in a controlled, inpatient setting. A specialized hospital unit will have established criteria for admission. Table 6.2 lists the criteria established by the Diamond Headache Inpatient Unit at Columbus Hospital, Chicago, Illinois.

The NSAIDs have also been effective in the prophylaxis of coexisting migraine and tension-type headaches, similar to their action in both migraine and tension-type headaches. These agents have also demonstrated efficacy in the abortive treatment of the acute headaches and do not have the potential for habituation.

TABLE 6.2 — ADMISSION CRITERIA FOR INPATIENT HEADACHE UNIT

1. Prolonged, unrelenting headache with associated symptoms (such as nausea and vomiting), which if allowed to continue, would pose a further threat to the patient's welfare.

2. Status migraine.

3. Dependence on analgesics, caffeine, narcotics, barbiturates or tranquilizers.

4. Habituation to ergots; ergots taken on a daily basis, when stopped, may cause a rebound headache.

5. Pain accompanied by serious adverse reactions or complications from therapy; continued use of such therapy aggravates pain.

6. Pain in the presence of significant medical disease; appropriate treatment of headache symptoms aggravates or induces further illness.

7. Chronic cluster headache unresponsive to treatment.

8. Treatment that requires co-pharmacy with drugs that may cause a drug interaction and necessitates careful observation within a hospital environment (ie, MAOIs and β-blockers).

9. Patients with probable organic cause of their headaches, requiring the appropriate consultations and perhaps neurosurgical intervention.

10. Severe, intractable pain in the presence of dehydration, electrolyte loss or prostration.

11. Severe pain in association with severe psychiatric disease.

12. Pain necessitating frequent parenteral medication.

Any drugs that may lead to dependency problems should be strictly avoided in these patients. Withdrawal from the habituating agents should be handled in an inpatient setting. Careful monitoring for withdrawal symptoms can be accomplished, as well as supportive therapy for the patient, during initiation of prophylactic treatment.

Finally, an essential aspect of treating the patient with coexisting migraine and tension-type headaches is continuity of care. These patients have run the gamut of physicians and therapies, and consistency in treatment is very important. Patients will also benefit from knowing that treatment is available and they are not alone in combating this syndrome.

REFERENCES

Diamond S. Head pain. Diagnosis and management. *Clin Symp*. 1994;46:2-34.

Diamond S. Tension-type headaches. In: *Wolff's Headache and Other Head Pain*, 6th ed. Dalessio DJ, Silberstein SD (eds). New York: Oxford University Press; 1993:235-261.

Diamond S, Freitag FG, Balm TK, Berry DA. Ibuprofen plus caffeine in the treatment of tension-type headache. *Clin Pharmacol Ther*. 1997;61:194. Abstract.

Diamond S. Migraine and depression. In: *New Advances in Headache Research*. Rose FC (ed). London: Smith-Gordon; 1989:291-299.

Feinberg DT, Diamond S, Dalessio DJ. Mixed headache syndrome. In: *The Practicing Physician's Approach to Headache*, 5th ed. Diamond S, Dalessio DJ (eds). Baltimore: Williams & Wilkins; 1992:138-145.

Freitag FG, Diamond S, Solomon GD. Antidepressants in the treatment of mixed headache: MAO inhibitors and combined use of MAO inhibitors and tricyclic antidepressants in the recidivist headache patient. In: *Advances in Headache Research*. Rose FC (ed). London: John Libbey; 1987:271-275.

Headache Classification Committee of the International Headache Society. Classification and diagnostic criteria for headache disorders, cranial neuralgias and facial pain. *Cephalalgia*. 1988;8(suppl 7):1-96

Kunkel RS. Diagnosis and treatment of muscle (tension-type) contraction headaches. *Med Clin North Am*. 1991;75:595-603.

Migliardi JR, Armellino JJ, Friedman M, Gillings DB, Beaver WT. Caffeine as an analgesic adjuvant in tension headache. *Clin Pharmacol Ther*. 1994;56:576-586.

Schuckit M, Robins E, Feighner J. Tricyclic antidepressants and monoamine oxidase inhibitors. *Arch Gen Psychiatry*. 1971;24:509-514.

6

7 Special Patient Considerations

Headaches in Children

Headache is a common complaint of children and adolescents. The headache may be due to a variety of causes, including migraine and tension-type headaches, as well as organic origins. As with adults, the physician must evaluate the physical and emotional factors that may impact on the headaches. The treating physician must also be aware of the various issues that influence therapy selection. In managing children with headache, the physician must be concerned with reassuring the parents about diagnosis and treatment.

Frequency of headache occurrence in children has been astonishing to patients and physicians alike. In Bille's classic epidemiological study of children in a Swedish community, 15.5% of the subjects had experienced a migraine attack before age 15. Another 15% of the children had experienced daily or almost-daily, tension-type headaches before age 15. The study by Linet's group in Washington County, Maryland, revealed that 56% of boys and 74% of girls between ages 12 and 17 had suffered from a headache within the month prior to the telephone interview.

Classification of headache in children is the same as that of adults. The headache history is the primary tool in determining the child's diagnosis. In the history, the interviewer should address questions about:

- The mother's pregnancy, the labor and delivery of the child
- The child's growth and development

- Episodes of serious infection (meningitis, encephalitis) and trauma.

A computed tomography (CT) scan or magnetic resonance imaging (MRI) should be considered for patients with recent onset headaches or in patients who have noted a recent change in headache pattern. Electroencephalograms (EEGs) have long been considered essential in the workup of the child with headache problems. However, this test usually will not provide any significant data. Many children with systemic illness will present with a generalized headache. Obtaining vital signs are important in the initial evaluation to rule out febrile headache. Sinusitis may occur in conjunction with allergies or upper respiratory infections. Headache associated with acute sinusitis is characterized by:
- Fever
- Focal tenderness over the affected sinus
- Elevated white blood count
- Elevated sedimentation rate.

Subacute or chronic sinusitis may or may not be associated with respiratory symptoms, and the patient may be afebrile. Sinus x-rays may be necessary to confirm the diagnosis. Complications associated with sinusitis are:
- Brain abscess
- Orbital cellulitis
- Meningitis.

Treatment measures include:
- Antibiotics
- Decongestants
- Surgical drainage, if required.

Encephalitis and meningitis should be ruled out in the patient with:

- Recent onset headache
- Fever
- Lethargy
- Nuchal rigidity
- Other central nervous system (CNS) symptoms.

Appropriate laboratory testing should be undertaken immediately. Urgent, aggressive antibiotic therapy is required in these patients.

Some children will experience headaches due to ophthalmic causes, including:

- Astigmatism
- Refractive errors
- Eye strain
- Squint.

Eye strain should be considered if the headache is:

- Localized to the frontal area
- Triggered by watching television, reading or doing school work
- Relieved by stopping a given activity.

These patients should undergo an ophthalmological examination.

Exertional headache in children may be related to a specific athletic activity, such as weight-lifting or running. This headache may occur once or may be recurrent. The headache is described as:

- Generalized
- Severe
- Throbbing
- Lasting from a few minutes to hours.

The neurologic examination is usually negative. However, if abnormalities are observed, further studies (CT scan, MRI) may be indicated. Indomethacin may be prescribed if the headaches are frequent and severe.

Trauma can be a frequent cause of headache in children. Similar to adults, the degree of pain may not be indicative of the degree of injury. During the initial evaluation, skull fracture or significant brain injury should be ruled out. Neuroimaging is an essential element in the workup. In the presence of subdural hematoma and the history provided by the patient and/or parents is negative for trauma, the physician may be confronting a child abuse case. Headache due to subdural hematoma is often accompanied by seizures and other focal neurological deficits. The treatment of these brain lesions is discussed in Chapter 3, *Headaches Due to Organic Causes*.

In children as with adults, headache due to brain tumor may be nonspecific in location. Exertion and positional changes may increase the severity of the headache. Tumors due to intracranial lesions are also discussed in Chapter 3.

Some headaches associated with hydrocephalus may not manifest until adolescence. For example, congenital abnormalities such as compensated aqueductal stenosis may not cause any symptoms until the patient has reached adolescence. Physical examination usually demonstrates:

- Macrocephaly
- Papilledema
- Sixth nerve palsy.

Neuroimaging will confirm the diagnosis. As noted in Chapter 3, shunting is usually necessary.

The typical patient with pseudotumor cerebri is usually an obese female in her teens or early twenties. This disorder is due to increased intracranial pressure without any evidence of obstruction to the cerebrospinal fluid (CSF). The usual causes of the disorder are:

- Menstrual irregularity
- Obesity

- Chronic otitis
- Medications, such as steroids.

As discussed in Chapter 3, the most evident signs are:
- Headache
- Papilledema
- Sixth nerve palsy.

Visual field testing may reveal an enlarged blind spot. Neuroimaging is usually negative and lumbar puncture will disclose increased pressure with normal CSF elements. Treatment consists of removing adequate amounts of CSF to normalize the pressure. Diuretics may also be used.

The onset of migraine often occurs in childhood. However, it may not manifest as a headache. Migraine is an autosomal dominant disorder with higher predominance in females. Prior to puberty, migraine is more prevalent in males. The clinical features of migraine in children are:
- Paroxysmal headaches
- Relief after sleep
- Nausea, vomiting and abdominal pain
- Throbbing, pounding quality
- Unilateral headache.

A positive family history is reported by 69% of children with migraine. Migraine without aura is more common in children as an aura is only reported by 17%. Several triggers have been identified in children with migraine:
- Anxiety
- Minor head trauma
- Exercise
- Menses
- Travel
- Diet (chocolate, pizza, cola beverages).

In children with migraine, the premonitory symptoms are similar to those of adult migraineurs:

- Pallor
- Malaise
- Fatigue
- Irritability.

These symptoms are usually followed by frontal headache, nausea and vomiting. During an acute migraine attack, the pediatric patient will often go to their room complaining of photo- and phonophobia. The child expresses a need to sleep, and the attack usually resolves in 2 to 6 hours. In children with migraine with aura, the prodromal symptoms are similar to those of an adult with this disorder.

In treating the child with migraine, certain factors will impact on the selection of agents in both the abortive and prophylactic therapies:

- Age of the patient
- Size of the patient
- Frequency of the attacks
- Severity of the attacks.

In children under age 14 with infrequent attacks, pain relieving measures should be employed, including:

- Non-habituating analgesics
- Antiemetics
- Sedatives.

For those patients experiencing more frequent attacks, prophylactic therapy with cyproheptadine (Periactin) or propranolol (Inderal) may be indicated. Children have demonstrated excellent responses to cyproheptadine in doses of 4 mg to 8 mg per bedtime. The major side effects of this drug are sedation and increased appetite. Propranolol has also been used successfully in children and adolescents with migraine. The side effect profile appears to be less with younger patients. It is contraindicated in patients with asthma. Depending on the size of the patient, the usual dose is 80 mg to 160 mg daily. Attempts are made after 6 months to gradually taper and then discontinue the drug.

Some children will present with complicated migraine, that is migraine associated with neurological manifestations. These patients should be evaluated for possible arteriovenous malformations (AVMs), tumor or aneurysm. Neuroimaging is essential in these patients. To establish the diagnosis, the physician should determine a family history of similar headaches. The types of complicated migraine occurring in children include:

- Hemiplegic
- Ophthalmoplegic
- Basilar artery migraine.

Adolescents experiencing an acute attack of basilar artery migraine may be suspected of using street drugs. The patient may present with a variety of symptoms which may be alarming to the treating physician:

- Episodes of altered consciousness
- Agitation
- Receptive or expressive aphasia
- Occipital headache
- Nausea and vomiting
- Vertigo
- Tinnitus
- Facial weakness.

The diagnosis can be established by determining a previous history of migraine or a family history of similar attacks. Neurological symptoms usually disappear within 6 hours. Prophylactic agents used with other forms of migraine are indicated for these patients.

As stated previously, migraine in children may not manifest as headaches but rather as acephalic variants.

In young children between the ages of 2 and 6 years, episodes of paroxysmal vertigo may occur. These episodes are brief and sudden, and the child is not able to maintain posture due to the vertigo. Due to the sudden onset and difficulty in walking, the child and the parents are quite alarmed. These attacks abate within a few minutes but are recurrent. Organic causes should be ruled out and the parents reassured about these symptoms. Cyproheptadine may be used successfully in these patients.

At a later age, migraine patients will provide a history of cyclic vomiting during childhood. These episodes of cyclic vomiting are associated with abdominal pain and are paroxysmal, similar to migraine attacks. The physician should rule out structural gastrointestinal etiologies and determine if there is a family history of migraine. Prophylactic agents used in migraine may be beneficial in these cases, including in the absence of headache attacks.

Cluster headaches rarely occur in children, although it may present as early as age 8. In adolescents, the initial onset of cluster may occur. Male predominance is evident in cluster headaches. Treatment would be similar to that of adult cluster patients.

Tension-type headaches do occur regularly in children. These headaches may be described as:
- Diffuse pain
- Band-like sensation (occasionally)
- Not usually associated with nausea and vomiting
- May be associated with muscle spasm and tenderness at the neck.

These headaches are not always related to stressful situations. It is essential that a careful inventory of the patient's family, social and school relationships is included in the initial history.

Chronic, tension-type headaches do present in adolescents. These headaches rarely occur in children under age 10. The frequency of these headaches varies from a daily pattern to several times per week or several brief headaches in a day. As with adults, the location and character of the headache vary. Nausea and vomiting may be associated with these headaches. The headaches are usually related to some type of emotional problems. Frequent school absences are typical, and certain questions should be addressed during the initial interview:

- Family history of similar headaches
- Parental absence from home (separation, divorce)
- Substance abuse by family members
- Over- or underachievement
- Significant school problems
- Previous emotional problems.

As part of the workup, psychological testing is indicated, such as the Minnesota Multiphasic Personality Inventory (MMPI). Intelligence and achievement tests may also be indicated in children presenting with school difficulties. The adolescent with chronic, tension-type headaches requires a multifaceted treatment approach with medical, psychological and pharmacological modalities. Treatment modalities include:

- Family counseling
- Individual counseling
- Antidepressants
- Biofeedback.

Acute pain may be relieved by simple analgesics, and habituating drugs should be avoided. Children with headaches have demonstrated excellent response to biofeedback training. These young patients are more open to learning new techniques, enjoy using the instrumentation, and have not yet adapted a chronic pain pattern into their daily lives.

Headaches in the Elderly

Headache is a frequent complaint of the elderly. Although many headaches start in the early adult years, the patient may continue to experience the attacks late in life. Other patients will note the onset of their headaches after age 50. In comparison to other complaints of the elderly, the frequency of headache does not seem to be a major problem. Actual incidence of headache in the elderly is inversely related to age. The onset of headache in the elderly may be a manifestation of a serious illness, such as:

- Stroke
- Temporal arteritis
- Glaucoma
- Subdural hematoma
- Brain tumor.

The need for a complete history, as well as thorough physical and neurological examination, is prominent. Patients may also experience headache onset or an exacerbation of symptoms due to medications used for medical illness, such as the vasodilators. Also, certain agents used for headache therapy may be contraindicated in concomitant medical disorders. Treating headache in the elderly requires comprehensive evaluation and careful consideration of therapeutic options.

The initial onset of migraine rarely occurs after age 50. Patients will report a gradual decrease in the frequency and severity of migraine attacks as they age. Female migraineurs will often report a dramatic decrease in their migraine attacks after menopause.

Patients with migraine with aura may note the disappearance of the headaches but they will continue to experience the prodromes in the absence of headache. These migraine equivalents or "migraine without headache" consist of episodes of transient neurologic dysfunction or deficit. A previous history of migraine will establish the diagnosis. The symptoms include:

- Scintillating scotoma
- Vertigo
- Transient global amnesia
- Mood disorders
- Cardiac arrhythmias.

Organic causes for these symptoms should be ruled out. Treatment measures are similar to standard therapies for migraine prophylaxis.

For those patients whose migraine attacks continue into their later years, the clinical presentation of the acute headaches does not change. However, special consideration must be given in selecting agents for abortive and prophylactic therapy of migraine. Agents such as ergotamine that have peripheral vasoconstrictive properties are not well tolerated in the elderly. Isometheptene mucate may be preferred for abortive therapy in older patients with migraine, although it should be used with caution in patients with peripheral vascular or cardiovascular disease.

For pain relief, the physician should note that a delay in the absorption of medications during a migraine attack has been observed in the elderly. The addition of metoclopramide with an analgesic (aspirin, acetaminophen or ibuprofen) may enhance the effects. However, metoclopramide has been associated with the extrapyramidal syndrome and must be used judiciously in the older patient, with the preferred dose at 10 mg at onset of the attack. The physician should also monitor the amount of analgesics used, asking a simple question, "How long does a bottle of 100 aspirin tablets last?" Because the nonsteroidal anti-inflammatory drugs (NSAIDs) may mask a concurrent infection, the patient should be regularly monitored. Also, if the patient is using the NSAIDs for migraine attacks as well as symptoms of osteoarthritis, there is a tendency for gastrointestinal (GI) complications, including ulcer. Routine complete blood counts should be considered to prevent serious complications of GI bleeding. Analgesic abuse may contribute to a rebound headache pattern, particularly with those agents containing caffeine. The patient should be detoxified from the habituating analgesic, whether over-the-counter or prescribed, before prophylactic therapy is initiated.

Elderly patients may be more susceptible to serious cardiovascular effects from agents used in migraine prophylaxis, such as the β-blockers or calcium channel blockers. There is also a greater potential for drug interactions in this group of patients, and the physician should use lower doses and titrate increases or decreases gradually. The tricyclic antidepressants have been used successfully in migraine prophylaxis (Chapter 4, *Migraine Headaches*).

Some elderly patients may present with previous histories of migraine in whom the headaches gradually diminished. However, they will complain of a recent recurrence of the attacks. The physician should inventory the medications used for concomitant illness, such as cardiac problems or hypertension. Agents such as nitroglycerin or Apresoline are recognized as migraine triggers. Indomethacin, an NSAID often used for osteoarthritis, is also known to precipitate severe headaches.

Cluster headaches in the elderly follow the same pattern as those in younger patients. There is a female predominance in patients experiencing initial onset of cluster headache after age 60. Chronic cluster headache is noted for its older age of onset. Again, treatment options are highly impacted by the patient's age. Because of the vasoconstrictive properties of the ergot preparations, the choice of abortive therapy is oxygen inhalation. This procedure has been detailed in Chapter 5, *Cluster Headaches*. Prophylactic agents, including methysergide and the corticosteroids, must be used with extreme caution in the elderly and require regularly scheduled examinations. Vigilance must be adapted with the use of lithium in the treatment of chronic cluster headaches in the elderly. Serum lithium levels must be performed at regular intervals to prevent toxicity. Drug interactions are also a problem with cluster prophylaxis.

Psychological aspects of chronic, tension-type headache render it a common complaint of the elderly. The most common cause of chronic, tension-type headaches in the elderly is an underlying depression. The daily headache pattern is similar to those of younger headache sufferers. Frequently, the patient will note a diurnal variation to the headaches, with the pain worse in the morning and evening. A sleep disturbance (in the form of early or frequent awakening) is a common complaint of these patients. They will also present with a multitude of somatic, emotional and psychic complaints (Tables 7.1, 7.2 and 7.3). The elderly patient with chronic, tension-type headaches may present with memory and cognitive difficulties, and some patients may be misdiagnosed with senile dementia or Alzheimer's disease.

The treatment of choice is antidepressant therapy. Selection of antidepressant is based on the presence of a sleep disturbance. Amitriptyline and doxepin have sedative effects, whereas protriptyline is indicated for those patients without a sleep disturbance. Two newer antidepressants, fluoxetine and bupropion, have been effective in older patients with chronic, tension-type headaches without an accompanying sleep disturbance and who are refractory to other agents. Trazodone is also effective in elderly patients with

TABLE 7.1 — SOMATIC COMPLAINTS	
Symptoms	**Incidence (%)**
Sleep disturbance	97
Early awakening	87
Headache	84
Dyspnea	76
Constipation	76
Weight loss	74
Difficulty falling asleep	73
Weakness and fatigue	70
Urinary frequency	70
Dizzy spells	70
Appetite disturbances	70
Decreased libido	63
Cardiovascular disturbances	60
Sexual disturbances	60
Palpitations	59
Paresthesias	53
Nausea	48
Menstrual changes	41

depression. The treatment of chronic, tension-type headaches is discussed in more detail in Chapter 6, *Tension-type Headaches/Coexisting Migraine and Tension-type Headaches*.

Headaches due to organic causes, such as temporal arteritis, trigeminal neuralgia, and postherpetic neuralgia, have been discussed previously in Chapter 4, *Migraine Headaches*. Any patient presenting with initial onset of headache after age 50 should be evaluated to rule out organic cause. For example, all patients

TABLE 7.2 — EMOTIONAL COMPLAINTS	
Symptom	**Incidence (%)**
Low spirits, sadness	90
Crying	80
Feelings of guilt, hopelessness, unworthiness, unreality	65
Anxious or irritable feeling	65
Anxiety	60
Fear of insanity, physical disease, death; rumination over past, present and future	50

TABLE 7.3 — PSYCHIC COMPLAINTS	
Symptom	**Incidence (%)**
"Morning worst time of day"	95
Poor concentration	91
No interest or ambition	75
Indecisiveness	75
Poor memory	71

over age 50 should undergo a sedimentation rate by Westergren's method to rule out temporal arteritis.

Treatment of trigeminal neuralgia in the elderly presents a complicated therapeutic scenario. The potential for toxicity associated with anticonvulsant therapy is higher in the elderly patient. Also, elderly patients are more likely to be refractory to conventional forms of therapy. Depression and drug habituation are common problems faced in elderly patients with these chronic disorders.

The physician treating the elderly patient with headaches has a dual role–treating the headache problem and managing the physical effects of therapy. An

elderly patient experiencing side effects from therapy may demonstrate the following symptoms:
- Easily becomes fatigued
- Exhibits altered sensations
- Complains of soft tissue pain.

Patient compliance is difficult with elderly patients, particularly the patient with depression, disturbed cognition or memory, or altered senses. These patients especially need and deserve a continuity of care.

Headaches in Pregnancy

Profound changes occur in the hormonal status during pregnancy and may be observed as early as 8 days after fertilization and may continue postpartum, until normal menses restarts. These changes in the plasma concentrations of estradiol and progesterone are quite dramatic. Subsequently, these changes greatly impact on the pattern of migraine attacks.

Pregnancy has been recognized as causing complete remission of migraine or at least a decrease in the frequency of the attacks. However, migraine can also begin during pregnancy, particularly during the first trimester. Tension-type headache may also be evident during the first trimester and is usually described as:
- Bifrontal
- Throbbing
- Recurrent on a daily basis for several days or weeks
- No associated symptoms
- Frequently mild.

These headaches may be due to various reasons, including:
- Stress

- Vomiting due to morning sickness
- Fatigue.

The treatment of headache during pregnancy imposes significant problems in selecting appropriate agents. The ergotamine preparations are contraindicated in pregnancy due to their oxytocic effects. Pain relief measures are limited as the NSAIDs (including aspirin) should be avoided due to their GI effects and possible bleeding problems. Acetaminophen may be used in limited quantities.

Prophylactic treatment is hampered by the effects on the fetus. In general, no prophylactic agents should be started during the first trimester. Treatment during the second and third trimesters should only be undertaken in consultation with the obstetrician. The use of the tricyclic antidepressants is limited to those patients who clearly require pharmacological intervention for psychiatric indications, particularly endogenous depression of sudden onset.

Biofeedback offers an alternative non-drug modality type of therapy and it is noninvasive. Methods used in this training have been discussed in Chapter 4, *Migraine Headaches*.

7

REFERENCES

Balottin U, Borgatti R, Zambrino CA, Lanzi G. Clinical characteristics and long-term outcome of migraine with aura in children and adolescents. *Dev Med Child Neurol*. 1997;39:26-30.

Baumel B, Eisner LS. Diagnosis and treatment of headache in the elderly. *Med Clin North Am*. 1991;75:661-675.

Bille B. A 40-year follow-up of school children with migraine. *Cephalalgia*. 1997;17:488-491.

Bille BS. Migraine in school children. *Acta Paediatr Scand*. 1962;51(suppl 136):1-151.

Briggs GG, Freeman RK, Yaffe SJ. *Drugs in Pregnancy and Lactation*. 4th ed. Baltimore, Md: Williams & Wilkins; 1994.

Burton LJ, Quinn B, Pratt-Cheney JL, Pourani M. Headache etiology in a pediatric emergency department. *Pediatr Emerg Care*. 1997;13:1-4.

Dalessio DJ. The major neuralgias, postinfectious neuritis, and atypical facial pain. In: Dalessio DJ, Silberstein SD (eds). *Wolff's Headache and Other Head Pain*. 6th ed. New York, NY: Oxford University Press; 1993:345-364.

Diamond S. Pharmaceutical management of headaches in the elderly patient. *Topics Geriat Rehab*. 1990;5:51-59.

Maytal J, Young M, Schechter A, Lipton RB. Pediatric migraine and the International Headache Society (IHS) criteria. *Neurology*. 1997;48:602-607.

Miles CB. Treatment of migraine during pregnancy and lactation. *S D J Med*. 1995;48:373-377.

Rothner AD (guest editor). Headaches in children and adolescents. *Sem Pediatr Neurol*. 1995;2:100-177.

Rothner AD. Headache syndromes in children and adolescents: diagnosis and management. In: *The Practicing Physician's Approach to Headache*, 5th ed. Diamond S, Dalessio DJ (eds). Baltimore: Williams & Wilkins; 1992:207-216.

Scharff L, Marcus DA, Turk DC. Maintenance of effects in the nonmedical treatment of headaches during pregnancy. *Headache*. 1996;36:285-290.

Somerville BW. A study of migraine in pregnancy. *Neurology*. 1972;22:824-828.

8 Post-traumatic Headache

The patient with post-traumatic headache may seem an enigma to the treating physician. Frequently, the patient with a serious head injury will not complain of any headache symptoms. In contrast, a patient may present with severe headaches following a minor head trauma. Frazee has estimated that 7,560,000 head injuries occur annually in the United States. Only 6% are considered major injuries, and 90% of head trauma patients survive. Approximately 80% achieve sufficient recovery to resume their pre-injury activities. Frazee also estimated that 44% of closed-head injured patients experience headache.

It is important to differentiate between:
- Acute post-traumatic headache
- Chronic post-traumatic headache
- Postconcussion syndrome.

The Classification Committee of the International Headache Society has established diagnostic criteria for post-traumatic headache. Post-traumatic headache is associated with a significant head trauma documented by at least one of the following:
- Loss of consciousness
- Post-traumatic amnesia lasting more than 10 minutes
- Abnormalities on at least two of the following examinations:
  - Clinical neurological examination
  - Skull x-ray
  - Neuroimaging
  - Evoked potentials
  - Spinal fluid evaluation

- Vestibular function test
- Neuropsychological testing.

Acute headache is determined by onset of less than 14 days after regaining consciousness (or after trauma, if there has been no loss of consciousness), and remission of headaches within 8 weeks after regaining consciousness (or after trauma, if there has been no loss of consciousness). The onset of chronic post-traumatic headache would be more than 14 days after the significant event and would continue for more than 8 weeks. Goldstein has indicated that the term post-concussive headache is distinct because a blow to the head does not inherently result in a loss of consciousness. He encourages using the words "traumatic" or "concussive" to describe head injuries that precipitate headache. It is important to remember that the post-traumatic headache, independent of the original cause, is part of a post-traumatic syndrome.

The post-traumatic syndrome is usually associated with:

- Headache
- Dizziness
- Irritability
- Lack of concentration
- Intolerance to alcohol consumption.

The origin of post-traumatic headaches as a pathophysiological or psychological response to trauma is a subject of much debate. Research in the 1940s was conducted on veterans returning from the war who had incurred head injuries. These investigators, led by Brenner, attributed the symptom complex following head injury as being related to:

- Specifics of the injury
- Personality of the injured
- Compensation elements
- Sociological determinants.

Incidence of post-traumatic headache was significant in patients with pre-injury neurotic or nervous symptoms, and emotional reactions to the trauma. Headache incidence was also related to laceration of the scalp. In the absence of coma or amnesia, the incidence of headache was lower.

Studies by Simons and Wolff revealed that post-traumatic headache could be attributed to excessive muscle contraction, entrapment of nerves and scar tissues, and dilated vessels. Acceleration-deceleration injuries may also result in headaches. Vijayan and Watson reported on a series of patients who did not report loss of consciousness but experienced headache at the site of injury and who suffered scarring and entrapment of sensory nerves. They concluded that headache could result from scar formation or direct injury and disordered regeneration.

Post-traumatic headache can present in many forms:

- Tension-type
- Migraine
- Occipital neuralgia
- Traumatic dysautonomic cephalalgia.

8

Post-traumatic, tension-type headaches may be the most frequently occurring consequence of head injury. The clinical picture of these headaches includes:

- Continuous symptoms
- Pain described as hatband-like, cap-like or pressure
- Not accompanied by neurological symptoms.

The patient may also complain of associated symptoms such as:

- Vertigo
- Lightheadedness
- Giddiness

- Anxiety
- Malaise
- Fatigue.

Head and neck injuries can occur together. The following injuries may trigger tension-type headaches:
- Sprain of the cervical neck
- Exacerbation of disc disease
- Exacerbation of preexisting spondylosis.

In the study of De Benedittis' group, they found that patients with post-traumatic, chronic, tension-type headache had higher scores on the Minnesota Multiphasic Personality Inventory (MMPI) test in the following scales:
- Hypochondriasis
- Depression
- Hysteria
- Schizophrenia.

These investigators did not find any correlation between the headaches and the patient's:
- Age
- Neurologic deficits
- Duration of unconsciousness
- Pending litigation and compensation.

The clinical picture of post-traumatic migraine is similar to that of non-traumatic migraine. Preexisting migraine can be exacerbated by trauma. Certain physical activities, although not considered traumatic, can trigger vascular headaches. For example, the "footballer's migraine" is precipitated by the heading of a ball in soccer. If the patient had no prior history of headaches, the diagnosis of migraine may be established by a family history of this disorder. These symptoms could be duplicated by the rugby player who sustains a blow to the face during a tackle or a hockey player who is hit in the nose during a check. Transient global amnesia may manifest after mild head injury and has been considered a form of trauma-induced migraine.

Autonomic dysfunction with vasomotor instability is considered the origin of post-traumatic migraine. Sustained muscle contraction resulting from the injury may directly affect the extracerebral vasculature. A high familial incidence of migraine has been demonstrated in patients with post-traumatic migraine. In children with juvenile head trauma, the following symptoms, similar to those of juvenile migraine with aura, have been observed:

- Cortical blindness
- Hemiparesis
- Somnolence
- Brain stem dysfunction.

In the study by Haas' group of 25 children with juvenile head trauma, 15 had positive family histories for migraine. They also reported a 12% incidence of transient focal neurologic abnormalities with migraine in family members.

Cluster headaches can occur after head injury. Some patients with cluster headaches will report an incidence of head injury prior to the onset of the initial series. The cluster headache occurring post-traumatically is similar in symptomatology to the non-traumatic type.

Following fracture of the jaw or facial bones with concomitant injury to the branches of the facial nerve, patients may experience post-traumatic, trigeminal neuralgia. These symptoms could also ensue after surgical trauma. As with other cases of trigeminal neuralgia, the patient will experience sensitivity to touch over the affected area and tenderness of the nerve may occur. Other post-traumatic neuralgias may occur, such as those affecting the glossopharyngeal nerve and the greater occipital nerve.

After head or facial trauma, symptoms similar to temporomandibular joint disorder may occur. Myofascial pain dysfunction syndrome may manifest in patients who incurred jaw injuries with stretching and tearing of the ligamentous structures of the jaw joint.

Vijayan in 1977 described a new form of posttraumatic headache–traumatic dysautonomic cephalalgia–which results from a soft tissue injury to the anterior neck structures surrounding the carotid vessels. The trauma was due to either blunt, non-lacerating or stretch injuries. The symptoms included:

- Unilateral throbbing headache (ipsilateral to the injury side)
- Excessive sweating
- Pupillary dilation
- Photophobia
- Blurred vision
- Nausea.

Between headaches, the patient may experience unilateral miosis and ptosis. The cause of the headaches was attributed to β-sympathetic overactivity. A clinical sign is the positive response to therapy with propranolol.

Neck injuries may cause headache after the traumatic incident. Pain may be noted in the neck, suboccipital and occipital areas. Acceleration-extension injuries, more commonly known as whiplash, are frequently the culprit in these headaches. These injuries are dependent on the velocity of the respective vehicles. Restraints, such as seat belts and head rests in the appropriate position, will prevent forceful hyperextension of the neck. The origins of the pain may be due to trauma of:

- Muscle
- Ligaments

- Discs
- Bones
- Nerve roots.

The pain may be focal or suboccipital-occipital, or radiate to involve all areas. Associated neck and scalp muscular contraction may precipitate the pain or exacerbate preexisting pain.

Post-traumatic headaches may also be associated with unusual complications, and the headache may not conform to a standard clinical picture, thus posing a diagnostic dilemma. Post-traumatic complications include:
- Daytime sleepiness
- Otogenic pneumocephalus
- Tension pneumocephalus
- Post-traumatic hydrocephalus.

The symptoms of normal pressure hydrocephalus may be present. Headache has also been associated with hematoma of the corpus callosum. Trauma may also cause:
- Visual abnormalities
- Monocular or binocular blindness
- Optic nerve injuries with anterior visual pathway damage due to sphenoid bone fractures
- Associated carotic cavernous sinus fistulas.

Traumatic dissection of the extracranial carotid artery may have a delayed manifestation as headache, occurring months to years after the original trauma. Symptoms include:
- Focal cerebral ischemia
- Oculosympathetic paresis and bruit.

It is essential that the patient experiencing headaches following a head or neck injury should undergo a thorough workup, with appropriate diagnostic testing. The use of computed tomography (CT) scanning, magnetic resonance imaging (MRI), and plain skull films can greatly facilitate the diagnostic process. Cervical spine x-rays may also be indicated. A family history of similar headaches should be determined during the interview. Psychological and psychiatric factors should also be investigated. Trauma can greatly impact on work productivity and daily activities. The MMPI may be an important tool in the workup and delineate the presence of anxiety, somatization and conversion mechanisms.

The treatment of post-traumatic headache disorders is usually similar to that of non-traumatic headaches. Management of post-traumatic, tension-type and migraine headaches utilizes conventional forms of therapy for these disorders. In addition to pharmacologic agents, the patient with post-traumatic headaches may benefit from physical measures such as biofeedback and physical therapy, including the use of transcutaneous electric nerve stimulators (TENS). A cervical collar and orthopedic pillow may provide some relief of the pain. Psychological counseling may be required for the patient with chronic headaches following head injury.

In treating the acute headaches, non-habituating analgesics should be employed and the quantities consumed must be carefully monitored. Standard abortive agents should be used and the available prophylactic therapies have been discussed in previous sections. It is essential that the treatment be individualized, with a comprehensive approach to the headache problem.

REFERENCES

De Benedittis G, De Santis A. Chronic post-traumatic headache: clinical, psychopathological features and outcome determinants. *J Neurosurg Sci.* 1983;27:177-186.

Elkind AH. Post-traumatic headache. In: *The Practicing Physician's Approach to Headache*, 5th ed. Diamond S, Dalessio DJ (eds). Baltimore: Williams & Wilkins; 1992:146-161.

Frazee JG. Head trauma. *Emerg Med Clin North Am.* 1986;4:859-874.

Friedman AP, Brenner C, Denny-Brown D. Post-traumatic vertigo and dizziness. *Arch Neurol Psychiatry.* 1944;52:36.

Goldstein J. Posttraumatic headache and the postconcussion syndrome. *Med Clin North Am.* 1991;75:641-651.

Haas DC, Lourie H. Trauma-triggered migraine: an explanation for common neurological attacks after mild head injury. *J Neurosurg.* 1988;68:181-188.

Headache Classification Committee of the International Headache Society. Classification and diagnostic criteria for headache disorders, cranial neuralgias and facial pain. *Cephalalgia.* 1988;8(suppl 7):1-96.

Landy SH, Donovan TB, Laster RE. Repeat CT or MRI in post-traumatic headache. *Headache.* 1996;36:44-47.

Moore K. Trauma and headaches. *Headache Q.* 1996;7:21-29.

Packard RC, Ham LP. Pathogenesis of posttraumatic headache and migraine: a common headache pathway? *Headache.* 1997;37:142-152.

Simons DJ, Wolff HG. Studies on headache: mechanisms of chronic post-traumatic headache. *Psychosom Med.* 1946;8:227-242.

Vijayan N. A new post-traumatic headache syndrome; clinical and therapeutic observations. *Headache.* 1977;17:19-22.

Warner JS, Fenichel GM. Chronic post-traumatic headache often a myth? *Neurology.* 1996;46:915-916.

8

9

Emergency Treatment
of Headache

Headache is the chief complaint on admission in 0.36% to 2.5% of patients in emergency departments (EDs). The incidence of headaches with significant morbid or fatal outcome is infrequent. However, ruling out organic causes of these headaches is essential. Once diagnosis is established, acute treatment measures and referral to appropriate specialists can be completed. Follow-up referral is crucial to avoid repeat ED visits and possible analgesic abuse. Repeat visits and obvious habituation problems will frustrate the staff of the ED and diminish the potential for recovery for the patient.

To adequately treat the patient presenting with the complaint of headache to the ED, the emergency physician should be aware of:

- Headache classification
- Appropriate diagnostic testing
- Available treatment modalities.

Headache classification is reviewed in Chapter 1, *Classification and Etiology*. The evaluating physician should be familiar with the dynamics of the headache history and the types of headache patient most likely to visit the ED. Although the emergency physician will rarely examine the patient with organic cause to the headache, ruling out these possible morbid causes is imperative.

Of those headache patients visiting EDs, 4.5% to 20% will be experiencing some form of vascular headache. Tension-type headaches are the most prevalent type of headache presenting in the ED. Narcotic analgesics must be totally avoided in these chronic headache patients. Table 9.1 details the differential diagnosis of the types of headaches seen in the ED.

The headache history has been reviewed in Chapter 2, *Diagnosis*. The interviewer in the ED has time constraints not experienced in a physician's office setting. Obtaining an accurate history may be difficult if the patient is in acute distress, and involving a family member or friend may be necessary. In the ED setting, it is essential to determine:

- Onset of this episode
- Any triggering factors, particularly trauma
- Presence of associated symptoms
- Any prior history of similar headaches or family history of headaches
- Previous and current medications
- Previous tests and hospitalizations.

The physician should conduct a physical and neurological examination, with the extent dependent on the patient's current status. During the examination, the physician should evaluate:

- Fundus
- Neck
- Throat
- Nose.

If the patient reports recent onset of headaches or a change in the headache pattern, the physician should be alert to possible organic causes. Presence of exertional aspects to the acute headache should also signify the need for extensive diagnostic testing.

A complete blood count is indicated if infection is suspected. If the test reveals a marked anemia, the physician should consider a hypoxia-related vascular headache. In those patients with status migraine (attacks lasting over 24 hours) associated with severe vomiting, serum electrolytes and renal function should be evaluated to treat complications of dehydration. Patients who are consuming excessive amounts of over-the-counter (OTC) or prescribed analgesics should undergo blood chemistries to determine renal or liver abnormalities. A sedimentation rate by Westergren's method should be performed on any patient over age 50 with recent onset headache or a change in the headache pattern to rule out temporal arteritis. Prompt diagnosis of this condition and immediate treatment is essential to prevent irreversible blindness associated with this disorder.

Neuroimaging is an invaluable tool for the emergency physician confronted with headache patients. The criteria for ordering neuroimaging are listed in Table 9.2. Because of the acute presentations of headache that are seen in the ED, these more rigid guidelines are necessary. If the headache pattern suggests elevated intracranial pressure due to focal lesions, a CT scan and careful eye ground examination are indicated prior to performing a lumbar puncture to prevent cerebellar herniation.

Lumbar puncture (LP) is indicated in those patients presenting with symptoms similar to:
- Subarachnoid hemorrhage (SAH)
- Meningitis.

Again, if a focal lesion is suspected, LP should not be undertaken until a CT scan has ruled out intracranial lesion. Xanthochromic or red blood cells will be evident in the cerebrospinal fluid (CSF) of patients with SAH. In patients with meningitis, the CSF will reveal white blood cells as well as bacteria.

At the ED, the most striking presentation of headache will probably be the patient with SAH. Usually, they will not provide a previous history of headaches. If they have a history of headaches, they will not have noticed a change in the headache pattern or difficulties with their treatment. However, they will describe:

TABLE 9.1 — DIAGNOSTIC FEATURES OF HEADACHE PRESENTING IN THE EMERGENCY DEPARTMENT

	Subarachnoid Hemorrhage	Meningitis	Temporal Arteritis	Hypertension	Migraine	Cluster	Tension-type
Onset	Acute	Acute or chronic	Acute or chronic	Acute or chronic	Acute	Acute	Chronic
Location	Global	Global	Localized	Occipital frontal	Unilateral	Unilateral	Global unilateral
Associated symptoms	Nausea, vomiting, LOC, meningismus, focal neurological symptoms	Nausea, vomiting, fever, photophobia, meningismus; focal symptoms, seizures	Weight loss, PMR, fever, decreased vision, jaw claudication	Nausea, vomiting, focal neurological symptoms	Nausea, vomiting, photophobia, phonophobia	Rhinorrhea, lacrimination of ipsilateral side	Multi-somatic complaints
Characteristic pain	Worst ever	Severe throbbing over area affected	Severe throbbing	Throbbing	Throbbing	Sharp, stabbing	Ache

154

Duration	Brief	Brief	Prolonged	Brief	Prolonged	30 minutes to 2 hours	Daily
Prior history	-	-	-	+	+	+	+
Diagnostic tests	CT scan 80% to 90%	LP (+), CBC	WSR (+)	CT scan to rule out bleeding	-	-	-
Physical examination	+ Focal signs, + decreased LOC, + meningismus	Meningismus, decreased LOC, irritability & rash	Tender temporal arteries, myalgias, fever	Papilledema decreased; venous pulsations decreased; LOC, CV changes	Nausea, vomiting, photophobia, phonophobia	Unilateral rhinorrhea, lacrimation, partial Horner's syndrome	-

Abbreviations: LOC, loss of consciousness; PMR, polymyalgia rheumatica; CT, computed tomography; LP, lumbar puncture; CBC, complete blood (cell) count; WSR, Westergren sedimentation rate; CV, cardiovascular.

9

TABLE 9.2 — CRITERIA FOR ORDERING NEUROIMAGING

- Clinical suspicion of cerebellar hemorrhage or infarct
- Stroke in evolution or completed stroke with emergency use of anticoagulants
- History and examination suggestive of intracerebral hemorrhage or mass lesion
- Acute signs of increased intracranial pressure
- Patients at risk for cerebral abscess but who require lumbar puncture
- Blunt head trauma with findings of increased intracranial pressure
- Depressed skull fracture
- Open skull fracture
- Penetrating head injury
- Head injury and Glasgow coma scale less than 9

- The worst headache ever
- Acute onset
- Nausea and vomiting
- Meningismus
- Focal neurologic signs.

The associated symptoms are related to increased intracranial pressure. With the onset of bleeding, a transient loss of consciousness may be noted. The emergency physician should be aware that the thunderclap headache can occur in patients with migraine or SAH. A 50% mortality rate has been reported in patients with SAH, and 50% of those with SAH who survive the initial bleed but do not receive treatment will expire within the following 2 weeks. Immediate diagnosis will increase the survival rate for these patients.

In dealing with meningitis, the emergency physician should be aware that this disorder can affect any population and is not limited to any particular season.

These patients will more likely present to an ED as opposed to the primary-care physician's office. The clinical picture of meningitis includes:

- Severe global headache, throbbing in nature
- Nausea and vomiting
- Fever
- Photophobia
- Stiff neck
- An alteration in consciousness (in some patients)
- Rash.

The age of the patient can aid in determining the causative agent for the meningitis:

- Hemophilus influenza—Ages 2 through 5
- Neisseria meningitidis—Older children and adolescents
- Streptococcal pneumonia—Adults.

Immunosuppressive therapy renders patients especially susceptible to these and other organisms. Immediate, aggressive antibiotic therapy is essential to prevent a morbid outcome.

The headache due to brain tumor has been reviewed in Chapter 3, *Headaches Due to Organic Causes*. These patients will rarely visit an ED as these slow, progressive headaches will usually respond to OTC analgesics and ice packs. Recent changes in headache pattern may alert the emergency physician to possible organic causes. Certain increases in intracranial pressure may exacerbate the headache, such as:

- Valsalva maneuver
- Exertion.

If the headache is accompanied by focal neurological signs, neuroimaging is indicated. These symptoms may also validate the need for neurosurgical consultation.

Headaches associated with brain abscess have also been described in Chapter 3. The emergency physician should question the patient regarding:

- Recent onset headache
- Recent or concomitant ear infection
- Recent history of sinusitis.

The pain will usually be apparent in the nasal and aural structures adjacent to the site of the infection. Brain abscess will manifest as:

- Headache
- Papilledema
- Other signs of localized traction and generalized displacement of the brain.

The associated signs of brain abscess include:

- Fever
- Leukocytosis
- Pleocytosis.

Certain generalities can be made regarding the site of the injection:

- Ear infection will usually produce abscesses above or below the tentorium
- Abscesses below the tentorium may cause hiccoughing, vomiting and occipital headache
- Epidural abscess due to a sinus infection will produce pain in the frontal region adjacent to the diseased frontal, ethmoid and sphenoid sinus.

The elevated blood count, in the presence of fever and purulent nasal drainage, suggests the need for CT scanning and possible sinus x-rays. Prompt antibiotic therapy should be initiated and referral to the appropriate specialist is indicated.

A simple rule for all physicians treating patients with headache is to obtain a sedimentation rate by Westergren's method on all patients over age 50 with recent onset headache. As discussed in Chapter 3, the need for early diagnosis and aggressive steroid therapy is essential in patients with temporal arteritis to prevent the irreversible blindness associated with this disorder.

Emergency physicians may encounter the patient with hypertensive headache. Diagnosis is confirmed by:

- Diastolic pressure of 110 mmHg or higher
- The headaches are worse in the morning and gradually decrease during the day
- Typically bilateral, although they can occur occipitally or involve the entire head
- Throbbing or "bursting" in nature
- Very severe
- Symptoms of catecholamine release may occur, such as tremors or palpitations.

These types of headaches may be a manifestation of another disorder such as acute nephritis and acute pressor reactions. Referral for follow-up is essential after the blood pressure has been controlled and palliative measures for the headache are employed.

The diagnosis and treatment of migraine are described in detail in Chapter 4, *Migraine Headaches*. It should be reiterated that an adequate history and physical examination can facilitate distinguishing migraine from a possibly morbid medical emergency. Treatment in the ED is focused on abortive therapy and possible pain relieving measures.

For the abortive treatment of migraine, several options are available in the ED. Dihydroergotamine IM or IV can be utilized. Sumatriptan SC can also be considered, provided that the patient has not used an ergotamine preparation prior to visiting the ED. The emergency physician may also consider prescribing the inhalation preparations of either dihydroergotamine or sumatriptan. These agents are described fully in Chapter 4, *Migraine Headaches*. The phenothiazines may also be used in the ED for migraine abortive therapy. In a recent study, metoclopramide demonstrated efficacy when used as single-agent therapy for migraine in an ED setting. Table 9.3 details protocol for emergency treatment of migraine.

Regarding pain relief, intramuscular injection of ketorolac 60 mg may provide rapid relief in contrast to other NSAIDs. Transnasal administration of butorphanol may be preferred to the use of injectable narcotic analgesics.

The patient with status migraine, ie, a migraine attack lasting more than 24 hours, may attend the ED to terminate the attack. Protocol designed by Raskin and Raskin involved intravenous administration of dihydroergotamine 0.5 mg, in combination with metoclopramide 10 mg in repetitive doses every 8 hours for 2 days. To combat the sterile inflammation believed responsible for status migraine, the use of the corticosteroids have been successful. Intramuscular administration of a long-acting preparation, such as Decadron LA 16 mg, may be utilized in the ED.

The short duration of a typical cluster attack precludes frequent visits to the ED while these patients are in a cluster series. By the time the patient arrives at the ED, the acute headache may have abated. Occasionally, the emergency physician may treat a patient with acute cluster headaches. The treatment of choice is oxygen inhalation by mask, at 7 L/minute for 15 minutes. Ergotamine preparations and other abortive measures are discussed in Chapter 5, *Cluster Headaches*.

At the ED, the patient with chronic headaches, either chronic, tension-type or coexisting migraine and tension-type headaches, may cause frustration for the staff and distrust toward the patient. It is essential that these patients be encouraged to seek follow-up care to prevent habitual ED visits as well as dependency on analgesics. Despite a busy ED, the physician must provide adequate time for evaluation of these patients to:

- Establish diagnosis
- Select non-habituating analgesics
- Refer to appropriate specialists for follow-up care.

Treating headache in the ED can be a difficult, unrewarding task. The staff may have a basic mistrust of the patient's motivation for seeking care. Unfortunately, there are patients who are drug-seeking and will make frequent ED visits to obtain habituating analgesics. In a busy ED, iatrogenic drug abuse is a danger as the overburdened staff will provide an analgesic, usually a narcotic, to free up the bed for a critically ill patient. Three measures must be employed in the ED for patients with chronic headache:

- Establish the diagnosis
- Provide immediate, palliative measures
- Provide referrals for follow-up care.

9

	Generic (Trade) Name	Dosage	Comments
PARENTERAL	Chlorpromazine (Thorazine)	1 mg/kg IM	50-100 mg every 4 hours, no more than two injections in 24 hours.
	Dihydroergotamine mesylate (D.H.E. 45)	1 mg IM	Up to 3 mg/day, 6 mg/week; may be used with antinauseant, such as metoclopramide (Reglan) 10 mg IM.
		1 mg slow IV push	Up to 2 mg/day, 6 mg/week.
	Ketorolac (Toradol)	60 mg IM	Up to 120 mg/day; no more than three injections per week.
	Metoclopramide (Reglan)	10 mg IM	Can be repeated every 4 hours, up to 3 injections per day.
	Prochlorperazine (Compazine)	10 mg IM	Can be repeated every 4 hours, up to 2 injections per day.
	Sumatriptan (Imitrex)	6 mg, subcutaneous	6 mg may be repeated after 1 hour, maximum 12 mg in 24 hours.
ORAL	Ibuprofen (Motrin)	1600 mg to start	800 mg every 4 hours up to 3200 mg/day.
	Ketoprofen (Orudis)	100 mg to start	50 mg every 4 hours up to 200 mg/day.
	Naproxen sodium (Anaprox)	500-750 mg to start	25 mg every 4 hours up to 1250 mg/day.

TABLE 9.3 — PROTOCOL FOR HEADACHE TREATMENT IN THE EMERGENCY DEPARTMENT

Route	Drug	Dose	Instructions
RECTAL	Chlorpromazine (Thorazine)	100 mg rectal suppository	Every 6 hours, PRN.
	Prochlorperazine (Compazine)	25 mg rectal suppository	Every 6 hours.
STATUS MIGRAINE	Chlorpromazine (Thorazine)	1 mg/kg slow IV push	Every 12 hours.
	Dexamethasone (Decadron)	1.5 mg	BID for 48 hours, not to be repeated in less than 3 weeks.
	Dexamethasone acetate (Decadron LA)	16 mg IM	Not to be repeated in less than 3 weeks.
	Dihydroergotamine mesylate (D.H.E. 45)	1 mg slow IV push	Every 8 hours up to 2 mg/day, 6 mg/week; may precede each dose by an antinauseant, such as metoclopramide 10 mg IM.
INHALATION	Dihydroergotamine	2 mg	One spray in each nostril; may repeat in 15 minutes, up to 4 treatments per day.
	Sumatriptan (Imitrex)	20 mg	One spray in one nostril at onset; may repeat within 2 to 24 hours, limited to two sprays per day.

9

REFERENCES

Akpunonu BE, Mutgi AB, Federman DJ, et al. Subcutaneous sumatriptan for treatment of acute migraine in patients admitted to the emergency department: a multicenter study. *Ann Emerg Med.* 1995;25:464-469.

Barton CW. Evaluation and treatment of headache patients in the emergency department: a survey. *Headache.* 1994;34:91-94.

Cameron JD, Lane PL, Speechley M. Intravenous chlorpromazine vs intravenous metoclopramide in acute migraine headache. *Acad Emerg Med.* 1995;2:597-602.

Diamond S, Diamond ML. Emergency treatment of migraine. Insights into current options. *Postgrad Med.* 1997;101:169-179.

Frederick RC. Parenteral NSAIDs in the treatment of migraine cephalalgia. *Headache Q.* 1997;8:219-223.

Jones J, Pack S, Chun E. Intramuscular prochlorperazine versus metoclopramide as single-agent therapy for the treatment of acute migraine. *Am J Emerg Med.* 1996;14:262-264.

Luda E, Comitangelo R, Sicuro L. The symptom of headache in emergency departments. The experience of a neurology emergency department. *Ital J Neurol Sci.* 1995;16:295-301.

Snyder H, Robinson K, Shah D, Brennan R, Handrigan M. Signs and symptoms of patients with brain tumors presenting to the emergency department. *J Emerg Med.* 1993;11:253-258.

Thomas SH, Stone CK. Emergency department treatment of migraine, tension, and mixed-type headache. *J Emerg Med.* 1994;12:657-664.

INDEX